RESTORING DIGNITY

RESTORING DIGNITY

The Struggle for Optimal Health Care in America

JOAN LUSCO GUGERTY

Copyright © 2015 Joan Lusco Gugerty
All rights reserved.

No part of this book may be reproduced in any form or by any electronic or mechanical means, including information-storage and retrieval systems, without permission in writing from the author.

The content of this book is for general information only. Each person's physical and emotional status is unique. The information in this book is not intended to replace or interrupt the reader's relationship with a physician or other professional. Please consult your health care provider for matters pertaining to your specific health and lifestyle.

ISBN: 1508647356
ISBN 13: 9781508647355
Library of Congress Control Number: 2015903266
CreateSpace Independent Publishing Platform
North Charleston, South Carolina

TABLE OF CONTENTS

PART FOUR

Dedicated to all who desire a health care system based on cooperation, understanding, and compassion.

Acknowledgments

M Y HEARTFELT THANKS go to all interviewees, who graciously offered their time and energy for this project, to the Institute for Integrative Nutrition® for their ongoing support, to open and caring health care practitioners everywhere, and to my family and friends, who give me their love and support.

PREFACE

L IFE CAN BE beautiful but at times very difficult.

Although the United States is the land of opportunity for many, there is a large number of Americans who experience their day-to-day lives through the lenses of sicknesses of mind or body, and that is challenging. Being in a state of optimal health from the inside out improves our experiences immensely and creates an environment where amazing things can happen. It is fertile ground for creativity, infinite possibilities, and life at its fullest.

We live in a country with amazing resources, stellar institutions of learning, enviable freedom, and infinite promise. Choices that each of us make on a daily basis determine the kind of life experiences we have. For many of us, the choices are limited by class, race, gender, environment, or economic instability. No two people are the same; no two people have the same needs or perceive the world in quite the same way.

As a child I was excited to be an American and to live in a residential community in Maryland with a backyard where I was able to play with neighborhood children safely. The United States was different then. I felt like I was connected to my neighbors, my school, and my church, as well as to my medical doctor, who had his office close by our home. Even then I was aware of being part of something important—something much bigger than my family or my small, individual life.

I don't want to minimize the social problems that surrounded me in my youth; there were terrible injustices being perpetrated by individuals, communities, and nations. However, in the midst of this, there seemed to be an invisible web that connected Americans—a union that I do not experience in today's world. The disconnection many of us experience today has been exacerbated by the technological innovations of the last twenty-five years. We are perceptibly more connected than we ever have been by cell phones, computers, and other technological devices. Yet there are studies that show that loneliness has become a serious problem for both young and old.

My culture is just what it is…mine. I cannot speak for other countries or even other states. I do not feign to know what most people experience, but I'm a good observer of people, and I know when someone is unhappy, disappointed, or falsely content. I examine life from the inside out; I don't profess to understand it all. But I am a very good student of life, and I have been blessed with a strong work ethic and an ability to make commitments, and I do not shirk responsibility.

The short story of my interest in good health began at the ripe, young age of twenty. I was looking for meaning and purpose in an America that was in turmoil over civil rights and the Vietnam War. I wanted to make a difference in a society that was struggling. I attended a modeling school to see what I could learn about beauty and confidence. As naïve as I was, at some level I knew I needed more confidence to feel motivated to pursue altruistic goals. I wanted to work with people but was not sure how that might manifest.

As fate would have it, the director of the modeling school that I attended was a seasoned professional and had been in the business for a very long time. All new students had their first class with her. I believe Ms. Walters was her name. I will never forget what she said in my first class, as I stood in front of a full-length mirror with the director at my side, looking me in the eyes in the mirror. Her words went very deep and resonated with me. She said, "Beauty is from the inside out." *Wow*, I thought, *what a concept!* As a very sheltered twenty-year-old, this was rather shocking. I had no sense of my power within. I knew I was in for more than a walk down the runway.

One of the mandatory classes in modeling school was a health class. The director gave a lecture on nutrition and good health, teaching that a healthy mind and body would make a more beautiful you. That one class had a huge impact on me, and I knew I had to learn how to be healthy from the inside out—both physically and emotionally. Although my modeling career was short-lived, I learned quite a bit. Thus began my passion for good health and well-being.

At this time in the 1970s, only hippies and the fringe communities talked about healthy eating. The US diet was perceived to be reasonable and healthy enough for most people. I might add that smoking was common, and although it had been identified as an unhealthy habit, our society was far from the condemnation of smoking that permeates our society today. Many of my friends and family were struggling with or not even trying to break their tobacco addictions.

Over the next thirty years, I worked in various medical institutions, hospitals, doctors' offices, and medical teaching facilities. I worked for a holistic physician for six years. That experience put me on track to learn more about nutrition and a healthy lifestyle and eventually to teach and coach others.

In 2006 I attended the Institute for Integrative Nutrition® in New York City, and I felt like I had found my home. Many of my instructors were world-class teachers, physicians, and internationally known practitioners. Through this experience, I learned as much about myself as I did about nutrition, coaching, and integrative medicine. I was in my element with some of the most positive and caring people I have ever had the honor of meeting.

Having worked in several hospitals and interfaced with hundreds of physicians and health care providers in my career, I learned much with regards to what occurs in health care in conventional hospitals, doctors' offices, clinics, and medical teaching hospitals. Although most of my experience was in administration, I had access to the entire medical culture.

My observation skills served me well in these experiences. For several years I was the coordinator of a medical-clerkship program in a prominent teaching hospital and regularly interacted with medical students, residents, and physicians. Most were caring people who wanted to make a difference in the lives of their patients. They shared their struggles and their successes with me, and I totally enjoyed working with them.

Patience is not a prominent trait of mine, but through the years I have become much more skilled in that area and in seeing the glass as half full instead of half empty. During the last twenty years, I have noticed significant changes in the health care system, although much of it is not positive. As the disease rates increased, I began to look more carefully at what was going on. I have read extensively about health, nutrition, and a balanced lifestyle and continue to educate myself.

Although I am aware that my life could end tomorrow, it is the quality of my life that I value, not the quantity. I am sixty-five years of age and in excellent health, and I feel great. Most people, including myself, want to have a purpose in life and want to make a contribution—these are what make life worth living. From my own personal experiences and those of others, I know that it is far easier to fulfill your purpose when you feel well and happy than when you are ill and struggling.

In my observation excellent health is not what is happening for our nation as a whole. What is missing? Why, with all of our great institutions of learning, have we as a nation fallen so far from optimal health? Why do we spend more money on health care than any industrialized nation in the world, with less-than-stellar results?

Many will say that people are living longer, and that is why disease is rampant. They state that many of these illnesses were undiagnosed in the past, but that does not account for the significant increase in chronic diseases, and it does not explain the steady increase in the obesity rate over the last twenty to thirty years. According to the Centers for Disease Control and Prevention, more than half of all adults in the United States suffer from one or more chronic diseases, and this rate has increased over the last several years, bringing with it increased costs in health care (Centers for Disease Control and Prevention 2013).

With all the billions and billions of dollars invested in research and medicine, we are nowhere near the top of the list of industrialized countries in regards to our system of health care. The last time I checked, we were ranked number thirty-eight. Our lifestyles have changed in many ways over the years. So have our ways of nurturing ourselves inside and out. I believe we have forgotten what is essential to maintain good health and to live fulfilling lives.

We can have the answers to our poor health in the United States and the exorbitant health care costs. However, a change in perspective is necessary to bring these answers to our attention. A health care system based primarily on economics and profit will hinder any efforts we make to create a more sustainable health care system that provides Americans with respect, dignity, and excellent health care.

Before we can even begin to make changes, we need to agree that people—all human beings—deserve respect and dignity as well as competent treatment in health care. When that becomes the goal of the health care system instead of power and profits, everything will change for the better.

About two years ago, I decided to embrace the conventional medical community as well as the holistic medical community and compile information about the patient experience as well as the health-provider experience in the health care system at present. I felt it important to channel my frustration with the health care system into a positive endeavor. Thus, the inspiration for this book emerged.

I realized that systems are made up of people. Both patients and health care providers are essential parts of the system. What they experience is a fundamental aspect of health care. The health care system may be huge, but every system has component parts that create an overall experience. It is important to consider these experiences when searching for better health outcomes and happier patients. The majority of health care practitioners truly care about their patients and strive to give the best care. Patients want to be healthy and happy.

What is good care? What is it that patients really want from their providers? What do health care practitioners need to provide that care? What is the hope for future health care? That is what I propose to begin to address in this book.

I hope to inspire those who are serious about participating in the creation of the best health care system in the world. Americans are capable of astonishing things. We are unstoppable when we have the will to make changes. With creativity, care, and compassion, we will birth a system that works well for both patients and providers and creates more positive outcomes.

INTRODUCTION

I AM WRITING THIS book because my values inform nearly every decision I make and most everything that takes priority in my life. I have struggled on my journey to learn how to take better care of myself in mind, body, and spirit and how to relate to others with compassion and understanding. My temperament is outgoing, and sometimes I am very outspoken. When I am confronted with injustice, I may feel anger, but primarily it saddens me. Then it motivates me.

Since I have more than twenty years of experience working with the medical community in various environments, I have extensive knowledge of the culture. I have encountered many systems of learning and healing that are extraordinary and others that are less than positive. Like everything else, the medical community is a mixed bag of good and not so good. But as it has grown in size, knowledge, and technology, we have lost something of real value.

The current US system of caring for those who are ill is less than it could be and certainly less than the citizens of this country deserve. Walking down any city street in the United States is an exercise in despair when one considers the overweight status of the majority of Americans, young and old. It has been said that the younger generation today will not be as healthy as their parents' generation because of their lifestyles. I agree we are on that trajectory. Yet as time goes on, more and more people are choosing another path.

While our government touts the importance of eating more fruits and vegetables, it simultaneously subsidizes the very food industries, such as wheat, corn, soy, and beets, that are used to create all the junk food we could possibly eat. Genetically modified foods (GMOs) are allowed to be sold as healthy with very little scientific testing—testing that is primarily done by the very corporations who create the GMOs. Studies that suggest the strong possibility of physical harm do exist but are ignored. The government also allows advertising to children and repetitive and very clever marketing techniques that encourage children to eat junk, as well as suggest that patients rely on drugs for an amazing life.

We as citizens need to educate ourselves, understand food politics, and be able to translate marketing techniques. Does anyone remember the tobacco industry? Yes, they are still around, but for decades they were allowed to lie to the public about the dangers of smoking. Is that what is happening with the food and drug industries today? Do the corporations have our best interests at heart, or are they primarily out to profit?

I'll answer part of the above question with a very troubling fact. I saw a news report recently that the tobacco industry is peddling their cigarettes to underdeveloped countries. Children as young as nine years old are smoking. This is outrageous, and it is hard to believe that any corporation would be allowed to perpetrate such deadly tactics. Freedom is not just about doing whatever we want, and certainly not when our actions have the potential of causing real harm to others.

Yes, we want to be free to do what we want when we want, to eat what we want whenever we want, but it is imperative that Americans be provided with factual information and that we know all the possibilities available to maintain good health. It is confusing to people when their government (USDA) touts the importance of fruits and vegetables, which are expensive to buy, but subsidizes the very foods used in the less costly processed foods and junk foods. There are over forty-five thousand items in most grocery stores, and much of these are composed of ingredients that are not real food but food-like substances.

There are hundreds of books on health written regularly that teach people about healthy lifestyles, yet US culture and the culture of conventional medicine are not conducive to a healthy lifestyle. Many people are overworked, underpaid, or unappreciated and dealing with stress at every level of their existence. When patients walk into their doctors' offices, they may be filed in, rushed through, and often not given the time they need to deal with their issues. This is difficult for both patients and practitioners.

My experiences with illness have been good and bad, and I appreciate all that health care providers have afforded me to maintain my health, but it is a constant struggle and a lot of work to maintain good health in our society. Why is that? With all our technology and know-how, why don't we have better health outcomes?

Listening to friends and family about their experiences with serious illnesses is eye-opening. I know that some of the pain, despair, and disappointment they have experienced are unnecessary. I know because I have had different experiences over the years in our medical system. But I had to work for it. I had to research and ask questions and insist on options. None of my good health came easily. But living with optimal health is incomparable. I would not have it any other way.

I believe that our society is ready, willing, and able to learn how to maintain better health. They are curious and frustrated with a system that does not always support their needs. There are many health care practitioners who have similar feelings about the current health care system and want to improve it as well. More and more physicians and other insiders of the current system are speaking out and writing books about their viewpoints. I have referred to some of them in this book.

It is time for us to speak out and empower ourselves in a system that too often turns a deaf ear to reason and to our needs. We as individuals may not be able to make the major changes necessary to create a health care system that supports patients and providers with the tools necessary to create pathways to optimal health, but together we can make it happen.

This book project is philosophical and value based. It is based predominantly on my experience and my interviews with patients of different economic statuses, races, and cultures, as well as interviews with health care professionals and providers, including physicians (both conventional and holistic and both specialists and generalists), nurses, therapists, acupuncturists, massage therapists, physical therapists, social workers, psychotherapists, and chiropractors.

As you read the following pages, keep in mind that all of the quotes that I use (although anonymous) are from real people who have navigated the health care system and shared their experiences, both good and bad. I wanted those I interviewed to be candid; thus, I am not using real names. Their anonymity, especially that of health care providers, allowed them to share more openly. All of the interviewees reviewed their individual interview narratives and approved them as accurate.

To be clear, I want to identify some terms that I use throughout the book.

When I speak of *conventional medicine*, I am referring to mainstream medical care by allopathic physicians and practitioners. This is the care most people experience in our health care system, and much of this care is covered by health-insurance providers.

Holistic, *complementary*, and *integrative* are used interchangeably when referring to health care that embraces the patient as a whole person (body, mind, and spirit) and treats him or her as a unique individual. It can include traditional Chinese medicine, complementary modalities used by holistic physicians and other practitioners, and modalities such as acupuncture and massage. The term *natural medicine* is similar to the above but would not include conventional methods such as drugs or interventions such as surgery.

Lastly, *functional medicine* focuses on the causes of diseases rather than the diseases themselves, works in partnerships with patients, and addresses each patient as unique in mind and body. These practitioners may include "genetics, environment and lifestyle" when making an assessment (Institute for Functional Medicine 2015).

Although this writing is far from all inclusive, it is my humble attempt to speak out and to give other people a voice in a system of health care that I believe has lost its way. This country has the ability to make the necessary changes, and we as citizens have a right to be heard loud and clear.

Maya Angelou has been quoted many times as saying, "When you know better, you do better." May this reading help you get in touch with your needs and desires, inspire more self-responsibility and education, and provoke a commitment to do your part to create a better system. Whether you are a patient or a provider of care, it is imperative to become part of the solution.

In his book *The Tipping Point,* Malcolm Gladwell suggests that small events create big changes. In his research he discovered that although the big events get the attention, it is the smaller events that make all the difference. Are you willing to participate in the creation of a better, more caring, and more effective health care system? Your voice is important.

Part One

The Journey to Now

1

EVOLVING HEALING SYSTEMS

Imagination is more important than knowledge.

~ *ALBERT EINSTEIN*

THE HUMAN BODY is a miracle. It is the most complex system that humans have encountered on this planet. Since the beginning of recorded history, humankind has been struggling to understand this magnificent specimen. There have been both amazing and life-changing discoveries over the many centuries since we began to record and study the workings of the body, mind, and spirit. Through it all, the curiosity and search have rarely wavered. It continues to this day.

According to Steve Parker in the book *Kill or Cure,* the history of healing and medicine goes back to prehistoric humans. Archeological evidence provides information dating as far back as thirty thousand years ago that suggests the use of herbs. These herbs may have been the first medicines. In Mesopotamia (current-day Iraq) about five thousand years ago, healing consisted of a combination of sorcery, herbs, and some surgery. It appears that, at that time, the common beliefs were in spells, evil spirits, deities, and the like. In that period religion and healing were merged together in ancient Egypt. History describes a medical healer named Imhotep who claimed great power and was raised to the rank of a god. His reputation continued on in ancient Greece, and he is credited with the quote "Eat, drink, and be merry, for tomorrow we shall die" (Parker 2013).

Although the Greeks borrowed from the Egyptians, they connected illness with the elements of our planet—"earth, wind, fire, air." Different fluids and organs of the body were associated with the seasons as well. This type of medicine was called *humorism*, and bloodletting was a common treatment that was used. Hippocrates, who is considered the father of Western medicine, wrote about the humors (probably with the assistance of his disciples) and made a distinction between healing and religion. He believed that ignorance was the cause of people's beliefs that the source of illness was demonic. He is the author of the belief that the first rule of medicine is to do no harm, and he is quoted as saying, "Wherever the art of medicine is loved, there is also a love of humanity" (Parker 2013, 22, 24).

In the Roman Empire lived a Greek named Claudius Galen who was highly instrumental in moving medicine forward. He had great influence in Rome and was considered one of the greatest physicians of his time. He learned from his extensive experience with gladiators, and he contributed greatly to medical knowledge, writing extensively. He was a physician and philosopher, and he studied pharmacology and anatomy as well. Galen expounded on the humors and suggested a correlation between temperament and physical health. He, along with other physicians of the time, used herbs and minerals for medicinal purposes. Galen also used advanced surgical methods (Parker 2013, 27, 40–44).

After the Roman Empire collapsed, there was a time referred to as the Dark Ages. This continued until the enlightenment of the Renaissance. During this unenlightened period, the Catholic Church became extremely powerful and influential. Healing became directly connected to God, and physicians were not credited for their work as healers. Although some laypeople were denied care for various religious reasons, those in the hierarchy were not held to those standards and were recipients of the best medical care available.

This was a time of witches and unrestrained religious power. However, people who lived in rural areas continued to use herbs and other natural healing remedies. Institutions that resembled hospitals emerged, usually initiated by religious orders involving nuns and monks. The compassion, cleanliness, and sanitation of these institutions were provided to many different classes of society.

In addition, the Catholic Church with its excessive power did not allow incisions and other surgical methods unless they were critical or were being provided for a nobleman. Ignorance prevailed, and people with leprosy were thought to be the living dead. This was not a favorable time to become ill or diseased, unless you were someone in power (Parker 2013, 52–53).

TRADITIONAL MEDICINE IN THE EAST

Chinese medicine has a long, established history and has been used for thousands of years. A Chinese proverb states that the best doctor prevented illness and that the inferior doctor had to treat disease. Much emphasis was put on maintaining a healthy, well-balanced body.

Acupuncture has its roots in Eastern medicine, and the pulse (along with other measures) was used as a diagnostic tool. Acupuncture opens the channels of energy in the body (qi) so that it can heal. Maintaining a balance in the body using herbs, diets, meditation, exercise, and other natural measures were basic treatments in Chinese medicine, and they continue today (Parker 2013, 64–68).

ALCHEMY

Alchemy is believed to have been used as far back as two thousand years ago. Its use diminished greatly after the Roman Empire fell but was revived later in Europe in the eleventh century.

Alchemists used their knowledge of chemistry to create medicines. Spirituality was deeply ingrained in the practice, and it was believed that a person's spiritual or mystical state comingled with other elements to create healing. The true alchemist was rare and considered to be gifted (Parker 2013, 56, 59).

NATIVE AMERICAN MEDICINE

Healers were known as medicine men or women or shamans. They were highly trained and greatly revered. Native Americans believed that healing of mind, body, and spirit was necessary for good health and dealt with illness in this manner. They believed in spirits and considered the Great Spirit to be intricately involved in their lives. Various herbal remedies were used for specific illnesses, and Native Americans believed that certain ways of thinking could also cause illness. Native Americans had many traditions that were important to them and gave them their identities. They were forced by the new colonies to end these traditions [although today many of these traditions are being revived]. They treated the earth with reverence and understood how much their lives depended on it (Parker 2013, 82, 85).

SCIENCE AND MEDICINE

During the Dark Ages in Europe, Islamic physicians continued the prevailing system and improved on the art of medicine. It was their age of enlightenment. In addition to the study of illness, there was significant focus on the cause of illness and on how to maintain good health. There were many writings on medical treatments and health. These are still considered to be important works in the field of medicine (Parker 2013, 103, 105).

In the West at the time of the Renaissance, medicine was more formalized, and medical schools were established, treatment standards were created, and physicians were elevated to a higher class. There were those physicians at that time who still relied on intuition and conversation with patients to gather data for evaluating medical issues, but they were not the norm (Parker 2013, 99).

It wasn't until the nineteenth century that the age of science in medicine truly emerged when microscopes were used to examine tissues and cells for pathology. It began a whole new age of scientific medicine. The modern uses of vaccines, X-rays, images of the body, and the modern study of the body's inner workings, came to be in this new age of medicine (Parker 2013, 286, 302).

The twentieth century brought innovations such as antibiotics, genetics, and fertilization techniques and sperm banks. There were also major improvements in the ability to lengthen the life span and in emergency techniques that save innumerable lives (Parker 2013, 286, 302–338).

COMPLEMENTARY/ALTERNATIVE MEDICINE (CAM)

After World War II ended and life became easier, there emerged a sense of freedom and change that allowed people to consider what they really wanted in life. The discontentment with Western medicine, with its focus on disease, medications, chemistry, and gadgets, came to a head. People wanted a more holistic approach and searched for answers in Eastern cultures. By the year 2000, more than half of the adults in the United States and Europe used CAM (Parker 2013, 320).

WHAT IS IMPORTANT IN HEALTH CARE TODAY?

It is noteworthy that Hippocrates's style of medicine is reminiscent of the caring family doctor and that Galen was ahead of his time by suggesting that there is a mind-body connection—a correlation between temperament and physical health.

During the Dark Ages, monks and nuns provided care to all people, including those in poverty and the outcasts in communities. The use of cleanliness and compassion brought hope in the midst of so much superstition and darkness in society. To this day this type of care remains an integral part of good health care.

The Native Americans believed in a strong connection to the earth as the provider of life. They deeply understood the importance of caring for the land that sustained them. In today's world, given the health problems from pollution and toxic chemicals, we can learn much from Native American traditions. Most of their ideas are embraced by holistic practitioners today but not consistently in conventional medicine.

Primary care physicians (PCPs) are frequently the first line of defense when we are in need of health care. They have more training in assessing the patient as a whole person, more often considering personal lifestyle as an important part of a patient's health. PCPs are in great need in our current system, and it would benefit all to establish policies that provide incentives to increase the number of PCPs.

Currently, there is little financial incentive to study to be a PCP. Too much emphasis is placed on specialties, which is reinforced by an insurance industry that reimburses specialists at a much higher rate. The providers that I spoke with struggle to provide the time and care required of a good PCP. They and their colleagues find it almost impossible to financially survive without buying into a larger group or health care system. These providers know what it takes to provide good quality, compassionate health care to patients. Many have been forced out of their private practices because they can only survive in groups or as employees of huge corporate entities.

Family medicine doctors are considered PCPs but have different educational requirements. They are similar but even more family oriented and in my experience have a more holistic perception of health. They see the individual patient as part of a family—all of whom very well may also be patients. They tend to spend more time with patients, and that provides a more caring experience.

Outside of the mainstream system is complementary and alternative medicine (CAM). The fact that so many patients in our medical system see value in CAM does carry some weight when considering how to provide optimal care to communities. People discriminate between what works and what does not. Most patients really want to get well and are frustrated when they do not. The information on CAM is voluminous but confusing at times. It needs to be organized in a way that makes it less complicated and easier to integrate into the conventional model.

The CAM organization needs to present the scientific evidence clearly and in a decisive manner. This organization may not have the clout of the American

Medical Association (AMA), but it has the support of more than half of the population of this country. CAM has a great case for improving the health care of this nation. There is considerable evidence that it works and works well to improve the health of the masses.

Nonetheless, Western medicine, specifically the AMA, still holds the reins for acceptable practice in medicine, and it has been very slow to embrace Eastern medical modalities. Those in this science-based system find it difficult to consider any treatment outside of the standard of care. This has been frustrating for many practitioners and patients alike who know the value of holistic treatment. Many patients know the benefits of CAM and prefer this type of treatment prior to more invasive treatments. Some courageous practitioners use CAM in their practices in spite of the lack of support from their more conventional peers.

Coaching has enabled me to learn firsthand how difficult it is for most people to make lifestyle changes. Patients need understanding and caring to heal, and my interviews confirmed my belief that people are not just bodies that need medicine or surgery, but people who want healing of their minds, bodies, and spirits. The holistic approach will bring great value to conventional practices. It is not to be feared and does not pose a threat. When integrated into our health care system, it will serve to provide care that more than half of Americans want and need.

There will always be people who do not follow the rules of healthy living, who are unable to follow the rules, or who experience accidents or diseases not of their own making. For this, conventional medicine is key. Caring for these patients is what conventional medicine does best. Holistic practices are complements to conventional medicine, not replacements.

Although many professionals in the health care system paint a picture that choosing care is an either-or choice between conventional or natural medicine, it is not the case. All of the patients and practitioners I interviewed expressed concern over their inability to safely choose care that is not the standard. The regulatory system has the responsibility to provide boundaries that are more flexible and inclusive of a variety of proven and safe modalities. As confirmed by all of my interviews with patients, no two patients are alike and everyone must be treated accordingly.

THE WHOLE PICTURE

Throughout history, people have struggled with illnesses and diseases and used their imaginations and skills to explore the mysteries of life and the human body. The wisdom of the ages is there for our comprehension and integration. It is not to be thrown aside like an old rag. Today's medicine is built on the foundation of the healers that came before us. It is prudent to remember their value.

I believe that we have evolved and are more capable now than we have ever been to solve some of the great medical mysteries. But we must not forget the wisdom of the past and be so arrogant as to think that we know so much better than they did. Yes, we know much more now about bodily systems, and technology has allowed us to venture places we never imagined we could go. However, we must build on the wisdom that was painstakingly acquired and make adjustments where necessary.

As I ventured into the minds and hearts of the many patients and practitioners I spoke with, this wisdom appeared repeatedly. Illness is not just a broken body; it is sometimes a broken heart or a broken life. Listening and recognizing the struggles of another person creates an expansive environment of understanding and compassion. And most of all it creates a space for healing. This must be understood as part of the equation when considering the future of health care. Today's patients and practitioners and those of the future will have it no other way.

2

THE BUSINESS OF HEALTH CARE

The problem of power is how to achieve its responsible use rather than
its irresponsible and indulgent use—of how to get men of power to
live for the public rather than off the public.

~ROBERT F. KENNEDY

YOU HAVE HEARD it said more than once…the days of the family doctor who did house calls are over. With the extraordinary technological advances, the masses of people being treated, and the lack of doctors to support those numbers, we have had to make choices. The medical profession today is far different from the family doc in the 1950s. Those of us who remember growing up in the 1950s had relationships with our doctors—they knew every member of the family as well as where and how we lived. When I was sick as a child, Dr. Max would come over and check me out and treat me in my own home. I was in awe of him and knew he deeply cared. It was a far cry from a doctor's visit today.

However, the path that was taken to arrive at the current system started long before my childhood. This has had both positive and negative consequences.

Institutions of healing have become more business oriented and impersonal over the last twenty years or so. It is a conundrum that we all face in the United States, and there is a clear struggle to maintain specific values in the US medical system. The current system's delivery and availability of health care have evolved significantly over the last one hundred years, and these changes are important to mention in order to comprehend the structure in place today. I will give a brief summary of this evolution derived from the Public Broadcasting System website chart at www.pbs.org/healthcarecrisis/history.htm.

In the early 1900s, physicians organized and created the American Medical Association (AMA). With this came a more powerful image and professionalism. In 1901 there were about eight thousand members; today there are about two hundred thousand members. With this transition, free medical services dwindled. There was not yet any medical insurance. As time went on, there was a shift in the status of health care providers, and their incomes increased as well.

Throughout the decades that followed, there was governmental pressure to supply medical care as a human right, but the AMA and certain politicians shot that idea down consistently.

In the 1950s health care costs continued to rise, and health care insurance was offered to those who could buy it. The federal government firmly took responsibility for the medical care of the poor. All the ideas proposed for health insurance failed.

There were huge changes to medical care in the 1960s, and hospital costs were prohibitive for those without insurance. There were many health-insurance companies providing policies, and this model sanctioned the high cost of care. Medicare and Medicaid were passed, and the government encouraged an increase in the number of physicians. Unfortunately, though primary care physicians are essential for good care, government actions resulted in a 69 percent increase in specialists.

During the 1970s and 1980s, the cost of health care was a serious issue, especially with new technologies and a hospital culture that reflected higher costs and profits. The 1980s delivered privatization to the system. It became business oriented and more controlled by corporations. Medicare was reformed somewhat, and caps on services were established.

The cost of medical care in the 1990s increased at twice the rate of inflation. Managed care assisted in keeping some costs down. Reforming health care was proposed and again failed in Congress. By the year 2000, 46,000,000 Americans were without insurance for health care. In this decade, HIV/AIDS emerged, and there were almost 140,000 people with only a 40 percent survival rate (Public Broadcasting System 2002).

In the new millennium health care costs continued to escalate. Pharmaceutical and medical-device companies greatly increased television advertising (making record profits, I might add). Medicare was viewed by some as unsustainable, and many employers felt weighed down with the cost of insurance and questioned continuing it in the future.

According to Steven Brill in his recent book *America's Bitter Pill*, the pharmaceutical industry has some very high profit margins. He points out that other developed countries outside of the United States do not have the same high markups. The regulations in other developed countries don't allow such high profits. Brill states that this is the case, especially with some cancer drugs. He adds that if US citizens paid what patients in other countries paid for drugs, the savings would be about ninety-four billion dollars a year. Big Pharma claims that the reason for the high cost of some drugs is because of the cost of their research and development. However, in his research with the US Securities and Exchange Commission, Brill found that to be untrue. He states that research and development cost pharmaceutical companies about 15 to 20 percent of their profits (Brill 2015, 234–235).

In addition to the horrendous prices that a hospital stay incurs, the cost of new drugs can be unbelievable. Brill writes about a new drug for hepatitis C that costs $1,000 a pill. Again, in other countries where they regulate the cost of drugs, this same drug costs much less. The costs of medical devices and drugs are not regulated in the United States, and these costs are hugely inflated (Brill 2015, 449–450).

One idea that Brill suggested as a feasible answer to our health care dilemma is to create a new system designed with patients' and providers' best interests at heart. He would like to see the independent insurance company's role out of the picture and the transformation of our sick system guided by forward-thinking individuals who take into consideration what benefits both providers of care and those who receive it (Brill 2015, 455).

As long as all of the interested parties have power in the transformation, it could turn out to be a good idea.

Another model that has been considered by both medical practitioners and the government for many years is universal health care (government-provided free health care for all citizens). This is already provided in the Medicare system for people over sixty-five and for those with disabilities. Universal health care has been adopted by all the industrialized nations in the world except for the United States. The idea was most recently quashed in 2011 by powerful lobbying interests, who helped craft the Affordable Care Act to fit their needs for power and profit (including health-insurance companies and the AMA). Why would the AMA resist a change in the system? Perhaps our current system is working well for them and they don't want to tamper with it.

There are some very vocal physicians who don't think the system is working well, especially when one considers the cost of health care, access to care, and quality of care. They want universal health care and believe it is the moral thing to do (see the website Physicians for a National Health Program [PNHA], http://www.pnhp.org/).

Most of the physicians and health care providers I interviewed want health care for all but have no idea how to make that happen. Many of these providers are very tired of the problems and issues that occur in dealing with private insurance companies.

It is noteworthy to mention the Affordable Care Act (ACA), which was just passed in 2009 by a slim margin. It was signed into law by President Obama in March of 2010. At this writing, the positive or negative outcomes of this law have not yet been established, although there are many positive reports from those who now have care. Negative politics abound regarding the law, threatening the good that would come from it. Time will tell.

Lobbyists for insurance companies and other special interests such as the AMA fought this law with everything they had and managed to make many changes to it before it passed. They continue to resist any major changes to the system of health care.

Since these entities are in the business of making profits, one could conclude that the insurance companies and possibly the AMA are not always working in the best interests of those who receive medical care. From their own personal experiences in the system, the majority of the patients I interviewed believe this is very possible.

In an article dated June 10, 2009, in the *New York Times*, it was reported that the opposition by the AMA would possibly be a real problem for those who would like to have the public option as part of the ACA. As stated earlier, the AMA firmly opposed such an option, stating that it was a threat to private insurers. They claimed that it would cause issues for employers who provide private coverage. Those who support the public option do not agree.

What President Obama and others believed was that the public option would provide much-needed competition to insurance companies, which would drive costs down. This belief is at least partially based on the success of Medicare. Although there are some issues with Medicare, few people who have it would complain about its benefits. It is common sense that if an organization does not have the responsibility to make profits, it can focus totally on the service it provides. This service has been a lifesaver for so many people.

What is so disheartening about this entire matter is that we are the only industrialized nation in the world that does not provide universal health care to its citizens. This is simply appalling in a powerful nation such as ours. The right to life, liberty, and the pursuit of happiness is impossible when people are ill and cannot get help. As their health declines, they become more burdened and unable to be productive members of society. Not having access to health care changes people's lives permanently when they cannot afford to be seen by a doctor. There have been many cases where illnesses and exorbitant medical bills have caused people to lose their homes and their livelihoods.

Moreover, it takes those at the highest levels to change a system as large as ours. It is apparent that on this point, the entire industrialized world is ahead of us. How is it that all of the civilized world and even some developing countries understand that, like water, food, and air, good health care keeps us alive and well? And they realize that to have a stable, productive society, the citizens need to be healthy.

I entertain the idea that our country is still young comparatively. The cultures of Europe, Asia, and the Middle East are ancient societies. They have evolved with a wisdom that we have not. Yes, we came from Europe, but like rebelling teens we broke away from our parents to go it on our own. In our idealized state, we wanted more, and in many aspects the United States became more—much more.

However, somewhere along the line we forgot our roots, original cultures, and beliefs. In many instances we see ourselves as better than others, as this superior and powerful country that is all knowing. It is difficult to admit our errors and embrace other teachings when such hubris exists in a culture.

In our journey to greatness, Americans have taken risks. Many of these risks have produced outstanding results. It has been a societal experiment that generated great institutions of learning, scientific research, technological advances, and a system based on capital. This is intrinsically good—but unfettered capitalism is another issue. Although capitalism has its virtues, its dark side is very destructive.

According to *Merriam-Webster*, the definition of *capitalism* is "an economic system characterized by private or corporate ownership of capital goods, by investments that are determined by private decision, and by prices, production, and the distribution of goods that are determined mainly by competition in a free market."

That may seem relatively reasonable on first glance, but when one considers a free market that sees greed as good, we have a problem. Wealth inequality is extreme in the United States, and the middle class has dwindled. The economic crash of 2008 is indicative of what greed in a society can do. And given the lack of restorative action and our apparent inability to learn from history, it very well may happen again.

In the United States, the free market has not proven to solve our problems with health care. In a 2013 report, the Institute of Medicine (IOM) noted that although the United States is the richest nation in the world, we are not the healthiest. Out of seventeen major industrial nations, we are ranked sixteenth for women and seventeenth for men in life expectancy. The United States spends more money on health care per person than any other nation, with disappointing outcomes. Even wealthy people have less-than-desirable health outcomes, mainly because of poor lifestyle habits.

The IOM relates this dilemma to inaccessibility or inability to afford care, poor health habits, and violence in the society, traffic accidents, and poverty. Environmental issues, societal values, and public policy are also contributors to the US ranking. Other countries have a more adequate safety net for their citizens as well. The one area in which the United States is doing well is intervention—for example, diagnosing and identifying cancer (Institute of Medicine 2013).

Many citizens expect the government to protect us from greed and corruption in the system. They believe that it is the government's responsibility to assist in keeping large institutions and corporations from excess and from harming society. Government policy changes everything.

If we are looking to an unfettered free market for a resolution to our problems in providing optimal health care, I believe we will be very disappointed. Our government needs to consider the needs of its citizens as well as those of the corporations. This has not been the case. The propaganda spewed out by the insurance companies and the powers that be in the medical system cause confusion and fear. Since we spend more than any other industrialized country in the world, our health care should be better, but it is not.

Referring back to capitalism, note that it works when there is competition. In the last twenty to thirty years, the competition has decreased significantly in nearly every component of our economy. Corporations are huge and gobbling up smaller institutions. Major corporations like MedStar Health are taking over hospitals all over the nation. Bigger is not better and certainly does not provide better care, as my interviewees confirmed. Huge corporations run as businesses, and most patients want to be treated with compassion, not just as customers.

Most of the patients I spoke with feel that as institutions have increased in size, the quality of care has changed. A male patient shares that "care becomes a commodity. Its focus is on the bottom line. The bigger the bottom line gets, the more impersonal health care gets."

A female patient recalls her experiences: "Regarding outcomes of my medical care, many hospitals and physician groups are run by megacorporations—they seem to hold our lives in their greedy hands."

As a professional, a retired nurse talked about her experience working in a corporate health care system where corporate offices determine treatment and care. She stated that she believes that the "fancy artwork and ambiance in a hospital costs a lot and that the care is not as good as it was." She continued, "It needs to be clean, comfortable, and organized—not look like a hotel. The focus does not seem to be on the patient but on selling. I am more concerned about the patient care, not the way the office or hospital looks."

There is, of course, the necessity for health care providers to survive in this new climate, and as one interviewee stated, "Corporations run a lot of hospitals, and certain monetary expectations are part of the system." That affects the quality of care as well.

When a corporation is very large, it is hard to pinpoint blame when things go wrong. It is my observation that this can be very convenient for those in the highest levels of the corporation. They can always claim that they were not aware and pass the buck to someone on a lower level. In my opinion, this merely creates a scapegoat and is totally irresponsible.

In 2008 the CEOs of some major banks and Wall Street firms, who were making six figures and in some cases millions, feigned ignorance when questioned on the recklessness of the industry. One could understandably expect that CEOs would have a better handle on things. But if they were aware, they are not telling those in authority.

Most Americans are aware that no CEO of a large bank or Wall Street firm has been made to be accountable for bringing down our economy in 2008 and causing immeasurable damage to the citizens of this nation. Our government exists for such things and is not doing a very good job at protecting us from these big corporations, including the entities that provide and manage health care. There is just too much money in politics.

As one physician summarized it, "Lobbying is corrupting the system. The FDA and government systems support the medical system as it is. These lobbyists move from the insurance company to a government job, and it goes back and forth. Totally corrupt." He added, "I'm an expert witness in a lot of cases where they go after natural-medicine doctors."

Health care is a billion-dollar industry. There is tremendous power in the hands of those who run it and a lot of money to be made or lost. At times, business as usual puts profits before people. That is just not acceptable in an industry whose main reason for existence is to bring sick people back to good health.

Moreover, I emphasize that although providers of care have some responsibility in the continuation of a system that does not work and that there are those who profit from this system, most practitioners do want to provide good care to their patients. As one patient said to me, "Many providers feel that they are in a bind and want to provide better care to their patients."

THE INSURANCE INDUSTRY

I invite you to read the book *Deadly Spin* by Wendell Potter, a once-powerful executive in the insurance industry. Unfortunately, as he states, "Perception is reality," regarding whether or not there is any truth to a statement of fact. He asserts that for the insurance companies, "it is all about money" and that the huge profits are always there for the stock market and for the snowballing executive compensation. Consider that while the CEO of Medicare/Medicaid makes no higher than $176,000 annually, CEOs of health-insurance corporations make about one million dollars annually when you take into consideration some very expensive perks, such as retreats in Hawaii (Potter 2010).

Moreover, according to the Institute for Policy Studies website, until the Affordable Care Act was passed, taxpayers were subsidizing these executives' salaries. In 2012 a large health insurer saved 1.5 million dollars in taxes through tax loopholes. In December 2012 after the ACA was passed, this tax loophole for executives was eliminated. The deductions on executive salaries went from 96 percent down to 27 percent—a huge savings for taxpayers.

In addition, the ACA provision for CEO salaries is being considered in Congress for application to all US corporations. That is very good news for the citizens of this nation who are feeling financially squeezed, especially since the downturn of 2008 (Institute for Policy Studies 2014).

However, one cannot ignore that the big insurers fought the ACA all the way. They made certain that they didn't have any real competition that would affect their bottom lines; they managed to mold the ACA bill more to their liking. A public option very likely would have lowered the total cost of health insurance by providing strong competition for the for-profit companies. The lobbyists for these companies did not want the competition of the public option and applied enough pressure so that it was not included in the final bill. These companies have very powerful representation in Washington, DC.

What the ACA also did for individuals with serious illnesses was to prohibit insurers from canceling people's medical insurance because it was costing the company too much money. However, insurance companies still hold the lives of many patients in their hands. It is not uncommon for insurers to wiggle out of paying for certain procedures ordered by physicians. Nearly all of the providers and medical professionals I interviewed complained that because of the power the insurers have, often they are unable to provide the care that they know is right for their patients.

Patients want their medical care between them and the providers of care, not the insurance companies. Because of time limitations and lack of coverage for essential consultations that determine the appropriate treatment for an individual patient, insurance companies actually block the best and most effective care available. When patients' illnesses progress, it costs more for everyone in the system.

Furthermore, because of a lack of participation from natural medicine providers in determining the acceptable modalities for use in patient care, insurance companies may not consider all options available to patients, limiting the ability of the practitioner to provide treatments that may provide optimal care.

INSURANCE CODING SYSTEMS

It is noteworthy to mention the coding system in health care. The most well-known codes, the CPT codes, are developed and owned by the AMA. CPT stands for Current Procedural Terminology, and these codes were created to standardize the language used to submit claims to insurers. This is, of course, very helpful in determining whether coverage is appropriate, but in creating these codes the AMA has become one of the main authorities on who gets reimbursed for illnesses and what gets reimbursed. It puts a lot of power in the hands of the AMA and the insurance companies.

The AMA makes a considerable amount of money from the use of CPT codes, money that they state is in part used to educate the public. The use of CPT codes brings in over one hundred million dollars a year (Medical Newswire 2007).

There are also ICD codes (International Classification of Diseases), as adopted by the United States, developed by the World Health Organization (WHO) to classify disease and mortality. This system is currently managed by the CDC, the National Center for Health Statistics, and Centers for Medicare and Medicaid Services (Medical Coding 2015).

These coding systems are not all inclusive but are two of the main systems used in medical care today.

In the 1990s a forward-thinking insurance expert decided to leave the insurance industry and create a new system of medical coding. I spoke with her about two years ago. She saw the gap in coding for medical practitioners other than physicians, as well as complementary/natural medical providers. Her creation was seen as a threat to the standard coding systems. The pressure from those in power and a lack of funding forced the company to reorganize and work with those already involved in coding in the industry. However, the CEO of ABC codes was able to develop a cost-effective system that embraces providers (such as nurse practitioners) who work within their scope of practice and provide less costly medical care than that received from physicians. The codes also encompass procedures and services provided by integrative and complementary/natural medicine providers and physicians (ABC Coding Solutions 2015).

These codes show promise when considering the high cost of health care in this country. They expand the definition of health care to include a much broader range of care than that provided by most physicians and health care facilities.

Although we do not hear much about innovations being made in the industry, there are many professionals working under the radar to create a more caring, equitable, and affordable health care system. Both patients and providers want that—they demand that. Many people are losing their homes or their livelihoods over illnesses and medical bills.

Business as usual is an affront to what the United States stands for. A for-profit system in which a patient who is sick can't get help or a skilled health care provider whose main purpose is to heal his or her patients can't make it financially is not freedom—it is tyranny. As a patient said to me recently, "Profit from sick people? Really?" What are the values we stand for in the United States? Is this what we truly want?

3

PERSPECTIVES ON CARE

The sole advantage of power is that you can do more good.

~Baltasar Gracian

On considering our current system of health care, one strongly empowered patient asserts that "the corporate model has not worked. Medical care should not be a commodity. It should be a right and natural thing that comes to everyone. Corporations own hospitals now, taking more of the humanity out of it. It is taking control away from the individual doctors. For good docs, that's a bad thing; for bad docs, that's a good thing."

Bigger is better? Ask anyone in today's society if they think bigger is better. Remember the economic debacle of 2008 to get a perspective on what "too big" can mean to the average citizen of the United States. Unless you are affiliated with a huge corporation and benefiting from it, chances are your response is that it is not a good thing. It is too easy to forget what is really important when the focus is on the bottom line.

When I speak of "bigger is better," I am not referring to systems like Medicare, because although Medicare is a huge system and deals with capitalists, its purpose is to provide good health care with a minimal financial burden on the patients. It can negotiate costs and is not in the business for profit. Its focus is to serve, not to make a profit.

A patient complains, "Unregulated capitalism is antihuman—no compassion, no caring, it's all about profit. It is not human or moral." Patients want to be treated humanely, not as commodities. One patient expressed this sentiment stating "The process is brutal, impersonal and tends to make me feel like a piece of meat, moved from place to place, with the doctor spending only a few minutes with me." "I am not just a car in a garage," voices another frustrated patient.

Some patients see the insurance companies as main players in the corporate model: "Insurance companies and managed care have caused all of these issues. It's become a business. HMOs are not planned on a human level. It is the corporate model, efficient and profit oriented."

Following this line of thinking, a nursing student shared that she thinks that the system "feels too impersonal." She thinks that patients don't always speak up because they don't trust the system and "don't want it [history and treatment] highly documented." She observes that "doctors work too many hours and a lot of them are burned out. The constraints of regulations they need to follow is limiting as well."

She continues, "In this country a doctor has to be careful with care. Procedures must be done in a controlled hospital environment, so doctors are not always free to use their skills in an emergency situation. Doctors are allowed to be doctors to a certain degree, and then they are smacked with rules and regulations so the medical system can be in control of the situation. Nothing invasive is allowed, even if they have their doctors' bags and can save a person's life." In addition, she adds, "Doctors are being sued right and left for every single thing."

Could there be a connection between the corporate model, regulations, and liability? Unhappy, frustrated patients will be the first ones to call their attorneys when there are medical errors. I have spoken to many angry patients— some have taken action against their providers, and others have been very passive and seem very confused over the poor care they have received.

Happy, cared-for patients may sue their doctors, but if you truly like your provider and he or she has treated you well, most people I've talked to do not want to retaliate for an error, especially when the provider apologizes and admits his or her mistake. The corporate entity cannot understand this—they approach the issue of liability from a business standpoint. They do everything they can to limit liability, but sometimes that caution is at the expense of good, compassionate patient care.

In US culture, especially of late, we have a tendency to perceive our country as all knowing and beyond reproach. Ask any psychologist how that presents in a patient. Narcissism comes to mind. Narcissists do not have the ability to perceive others' feelings, nor do they care about those feelings. Their pleasure and satisfaction are all that counts.

The health care system of today, as well as many other large conglomerates that have arisen over the last twenty years, appears to have lost sight of what people really want and need. Unless patients are independently wealthy and are able to pay out of pocket for all of their health care needs, the knowledge that a serious illness could threaten their safety and security is always in the backs of their minds. For-profit corporations must make a profit—it is really their main job. That is not good for the patient, as is stated in many different ways in this writing.

This negatively affects the providers of care as well. If a provider of care has to constantly be concerned and pressured to meet the bottom line to do his or her job and survive in the field, he or she may lose sight of what is truly valuable in healing. When a doctor is presented with a patient's illness, it is quite possible that it is not the next high-tech procedure or the next new medication that is needed. Taking time with the patient instead of working to stay within time constraints has a better chance of producing good outcomes—ones that are best for the individual patient being treated.

Recently, I heard a physician mention the franchise Massage Envy. This entity provides massages to multitudes at a very low cost. As it turns out, these highly trained therapists make about seventeen dollars an hour. That is where health becomes a commodity. I was trained in massage. It is hard, physical work but can be a very healing modality for those whose stress or pain lessens their quality of life. These small factories of massage diminish the value of the service when offered for so little compensation. If massage were considered to be within the standard of care by mainstream medicine, it would be more accessible to patients who would benefit from the treatment, and the massage therapists would earn a more reasonable wage.

In addition, minimal compensation is becoming the standard for many physicians and practitioners all over the country. To remain financially viable, many must work for large institutions as employees. This, of course, limits the amount of care and the type of care available to patients. It's a one-size-fits-all mind-set. The bigger and more powerful the organization becomes, the more obscure the individual needs of each patient. My interviews are reflections of the commodity mind-set.

To contrast that situation, let's take a moment to consider the salaries for the CEOs of these huge hospital conglomerates. According to the IRS, for 2012 the salaries averaged $500,000, with the top salary at $2,300,000. The president of the United States makes $400,000. I can't imagine their jobs are any more difficult than his. As salaries are forced down for the physicians, nurses, technicians, and remaining staff who make the hospital systems work, those at the top are demanding higher and higher salaries. This is a big problem and will definitely have negative results in overall health care in the United States. Those at the top set the tone for the values of the company.

Bigger is better? Unless you are affiliated with a huge corporation and benefiting from it, chances are your response is "absolutely not!" Individualized care has suffered greatly. The bottom line steers major decisions in these huge corporations—they have stockholders who they have a responsibility to.

When government policy is set, it makes a difference, and the laws that govern monopolies have not been enforced, or they are very lax. One after another, large corporations buy smaller ones, bigger banks take over smaller ones, or megacorporations run many hospitals. The customer or patient gets the bad end of the deal in these situations. The corporations bow to their stakeholders instead of making the needs of the individual customer or patient primary. This cannot and will not produce efficiency, and it will not promote the optimal health care system.

Don't get me wrong…there are many compassionate practitioners, but when doctors are limited in their ability to provide the care patients need and are overworked and underpaid, it becomes more difficult to continue to give as is desired.

It is common knowledge that stress decreases efficiency. Research is very clear on this. Some stress is motivating, but that is good stress. When it becomes too much, as has become epidemic in this country, the stress is no longer productive and often has a negative impact on the person emotionally and physically. This can produce low morale in any organization.

Out of the fifty interviews I conducted, it was nearly unanimous that the US health care system needs to be fixed. Most interviewees felt that all people should have access to good medical care. One stated clearly that "everyone in our country should have access to medical care and never be turned away." Although most people agree that some care in the United States is superior, many believe it is much too expensive. That in itself makes it inaccessible to many people in this country. Patients and nearly all providers do not want medical care to be all about money. As one patient stated, "Too little value is on human beings. It needs to be about human life." The quality of human life must be made more valuable than profits.

It appears what is missing in our system of health care and reimbursement for medical care is the concept of working together. It's as if insurance companies see people with health issues as liabilities and those who don't submit claims as assets. Do some providers see sick patients as customers as well as individuals who deserve respect? Is there a lack of humanity in these processes? Are those making health care decisions able to consider the individual challenges of patients and how to best support them?

In the book *The American Health Care Paradox*, authors Elizabeth H. Bradley and Lauren A. Taylor analyzed other health care systems. They reported that Scandinavian health care systems and their patient outcomes are far better than the US system of health. They spend almost half of what we spend on health care, and 100 percent of the population has free medical care. The reason the authors dealt with the particular countries in the book is because of the similarities in values to those of Americans.

There are areas, however, where our values differ. Although we in the United States have similar desires to Scandinavian countries regarding freedom and specific standards of living, we differ in a sense of community and mutual responsibility of both government and citizenry. Both citizens and governments place a strong emphasis on the common good.

Scandinavian governments provide free health care and education, as well as monetary support when necessary, to all their citizens. They expect that all citizens, regardless of income, will accept these services when needed. In return, all citizens have the responsibility to work, and the government supports them in different ways to afford them the opportunity to fulfill that responsibility. It is mutual respect on both sides. There is no name-calling or demonizing groups of citizens or government.

Those who absolutely cannot work are taken care of, and this necessity is not considered to be shameful, unlike in the United States, where people who don't work are automatically considered lazy and less than worthy. Moreover, Scandinavian governments provide a variety of health care modalities for treatment, leaving citizens with the freedom to choose the specific care they need and desire.

In addition, the social aspects of Scandinavian society are taken into consideration when determining the needs of citizens. The government considers a safe home, adequate support in the home (home-care workers when ill), and a healthy lifestyle as part of the equation when determining what an individual needs to improve his or her health and to return to being a productive member of society (Taylor and Bradley 2013).

In my view, what this type of system does is encourages patients to focus on their individual needs, choose what is best for them, and become partners in returning to health without relying heavily on their physicians or practitioners. As a coach I find this acceptance of responsibility for one's own health to be very empowering to patients. This shift would require that providers and patients work as partners. I believe that this general attitude alone would greatly improve health outcomes in this nation.

In addition, what improves overall health status is to have access to care. The lack of access to health care in the United States is at least partially responsible for the cost of our care and the overall quality of the health of our citizens. When patients ignore symptoms of illnesses because they can't afford to get medical treatment, often illnesses progress to diseases, which are very costly to the system and costly to patients' well-being and independence. When individuals become too sick to work, they then need more assistance from the government in the way of food stamps and unemployment insurance. It is a vicious cycle.

This is about values. It is about what is most important in our society. As I mentioned in my discussion of my own childhood experience, the connection to other citizens and the feeling of being part of a united group of states has all but vanished. We don't make choices knowing that we are all in this together. Our culture has made a major detour in this area and not to the betterment of US society. In a self-proclaimed, predominantly moral nation, the us-against-them mentality leaves us feeling isolated, fearful, and defensive. That is not conducive to true US values, to peace of mind, or to strengthening our nation. I believe the United States can do better.

What is lost here is what is for the common good of all involved. Scandinavia has the perspective that when the common good is the highest value, everyone benefits. In the United States, we were once seen as the country whose Statue of Liberty welcomed immigrants: "Give me your tired, your poor, your huddled masses yearning to breathe free." We have seriously strayed from our roots. I personally believe greed and fear have taken over our society.

This book is not meant to address economic issues, but one cannot talk about health care and the cost of health care without mentioning them. We live in a society today where the rich are getting richer, while a good percentage of our citizens cannot even pay their bills, especially huge medical bills. The cry for the common good is getting louder but has not yet been heard by those in power—and neither has the cry for a more caring health care system.

This is a critical time in health care. The overall poor health of our citizens will eventually make it impossible for the current system to manage. Things have to change, and they will. It is only a matter of time.

PART TWO

WHAT PATIENTS REALLY WANT

4

THE ART OF LISTENING

The heart has reasons which reason knows nothing of.

~*BLAISE PASCAL*

THERE ARE MANY experiences in life where we feel vulnerable, but perhaps none as frightening as being in the care of a medical professional when we are faced with illnesses. One patient stated, "I want my provider to be empathetic and listen to me...I feel weak and vulnerable and feel that I'm putting my life in their hands." In my research, it was no surprise that the number one desire of patients being treated in doctors' offices or any health care facilities is to be seen and heard. Although health care professionals may be provided some training in this area, it is lacking. The large majority of my interview participants confirm that.

Patients want a physician with a caring attitude—someone who is able to see the patient as an individual with his or her own needs, desires, stressors, and life situations. Many patients feel there is a lack of empathy and reverence for life on the part of most providers. I heard comments such as, "[Office visits are] usually like herding sheep in and out," "The provider needs to be able to put him or herself in my shoes," "If the provider listened more, they would get more clues as to what might be wrong," "I think a good provider gets to know you," and "I want the health care practitioner to ask me questions that are not from a formula, listen and analyze possibilities, and not make decisions just based on the facts entered in my file."

A male physician stated that, "You must listen to patients to get a good history. I have found that the patient knows their own history better than the doctor. It is very important for the patient to be able to tell their story." Many patients affirmed this—they want doctors to ask questions about their individual lives to put medical issues into the context of particular lifestyles. Repeatedly, patients voiced their concerns about not being heard by their health care providers. A female health care provider told me that over the many years of practice, she has been told by her patients repeatedly that "no one [health care provider] listens to me." This provider shared that, although it may hurt her bottom line, she gives her patients time to talk before any treatment is given.

The need to be listened to was not age or gender specific among the interviewees, although more women than men voiced their concern—from the age of twenty-seven to seventy-seven, patients want their health care practitioners to listen to their concerns and see the entire picture. They do not want to be perceived as diseases, numbers, or cases, but as individuals. People said, "I want the health care practitioner to know me well so they can make good decisions. It's very important for them to listen to my concerns," "A doctor has the responsibility of listening to you and hearing what you are saying," "They need to show more heart," and "I don't want to be placated." Patients want to be accepted for who they are: "They want to be validated and free from judgment." A patient can be given instructions and spoken to candidly without judgment.

Listening is an art. It is a learned behavior. It does not come naturally to everyone. If you have not been deeply listened to in your life or have not been trained to listen deeply, you will not be able to provide that service to patients. It is that simple. Putting aside all opinions and beliefs while the patient speaks can be challenging. It is very difficult to encourage patients to share their thoughts in a health care system that allows little time for an office visit. However, it cannot be emphasized enough. Patients want to be heard, and being listened to improves their experiences. In a society replete with stress, this is a great gift to any patient. It improves the patient-provider relationship when the listening component is part of a patient's overall experience in health care: "Practitioners need to learn how to have eye contact and give meaningful feedback—to stay present with the patient."

David Augsburger, a senior professor of pastoral care at Fuller Theological Seminary, is quoted as saying, "Being listened to is so close to being loved that most people cannot tell the difference." I am not suggesting that providers make their patients feel loved. What I am saying is that when patients feel listened to, they are more likely to feel that the provider is caring, so they will be more open, trusting, and honest. All the health care providers I spoke with wanted that openness and honesty from patients in order to have the necessary information and provide the best care.

It is well known that stress is a big concern in our society. Stress has been associated with every major disease in the United States. Good stress is not the culprit; chronic stress is, and it has become the norm for many people in our society. We all need a certain amount of stress to be motivated. But chronic stress over time keeps us in a state of fight or flight, placing a huge burden on the body. In the book *Stress Free for Good,* Stanford University researchers Dr. Fred Luskin and Dr. Kenneth Pelletier state that "stress lowers the effectiveness of the immune system, raises blood pressure, causes the heart rate to increase, the stomach to tighten and narrows thinking." In the United States, there is a major movement in yoga, meditation, and other stress-management tools to deal with the stress epidemic.

We know that stress is a major problem, but how does stress management relate to listening skills? There is a connection. Doctors Luskin and Pelletier extensively studied stress and effective ways to manage it. Many of the tools they teach relate to how people think and perceive their realities. One of the life skills was to teach people experiencing the stress response to visualize an act of kindness done for them. Using this skill, people fully relaxed in about six seconds. In that state of mind, the body realizes that there is no danger. Perception matters.

When patients seek out physicians or other health care providers to assist with medical problems, they can be made to relax and feel that all is well—or patients can have an experience where they feel disconnected and frightened. The providers I interviewed want the kind of experience that is conducive to healing. They care about their patients, and they want them to get well. A relaxed, open, and trusting patient is more likely to satisfy that requirement.

As a public speaker, I know how to connect with an audience. It is comparable to connecting with an individual on a one-to-one basis. That connection can be made in a moment when skillfully done. Making eye contact with different audience members, smiling, and engaging them in the process are all essential components of an excellent speech. Each member of the audience must feel that you are speaking to him or her individually. It brings the audience into the story, keeps them interested, and encourages them to take what they are hearing very seriously. Some speeches are interactive. That is when the audience really comes alive.

I would suggest that this type of scenario will occur in a doctor's office only when the provider of care sees the patient as his or her equal—another human face with all the frailties that are part of being human. When patients see their health care providers as equals but with skills in the areas of expertise that they are in need of, it is far easier for patients to respect and honor the treatment plans given. Patients do not want to be talked down to or patronized. Although some patients do want the provider to simply tell them what to do, in questioning further I found that these patients also want to know that the provider cares about them as individuals. Another desire of patients is for the provider to earnestly say, "How are you?" or just to remember something about them and ask about it. Patients feel vulnerable and are searching for connection and caring.

Engaging their patients is one of the most efficient ways for providers to create environments of trust. An experienced physician told me that he can look into the patients' eyes and know when they will not follow his treatment plan. At that point, it becomes essential to engage the patient and ask the hard questions. Many providers state they don't have the time or don't even consider it. I suggest a provider can't afford not to ask questions of the patient.

When providers do not know their patients, their treatments may not work for many different reasons. There might be pieces of personal information about patients' lifestyles that would change entire treatment plans or make it impossible for patients to follow through. Passive patients share that they are frustrated with their doctors and often don't get the care they need. Open communication between providers and patients is essential for good care. As a coach, I know that asking the right questions is invaluable in getting to know what a client really needs. One male participant explained it like this: "He or she [health care provider] listens carefully to the reason for my visit and elicits additional information that a nonexpert might not realize is pertinent." The patient does not always realize what information is helpful in acquiring the best medical treatment. Some patients will not offer any information unless asked and clearly want the health care provider to ask pertinent questions.

The perfect interaction with the provider might look like this: The provider is present with you in the moment, not multitasking; he or she makes eye contact, actively listens, and gathers the information in a caring manner. He or she asks questions that encourage you to share pertinent information in your life. After listening carefully, the provider uses not just his or her intellect but also his or her gut feelings for answers to your medical issues. Adequate time and care is given as needed; you do not feel rushed. You feel like there is a connection between you and the health care provider. He or she listens to your personal life issues and sees those as part of the equation. He or she does not perceive you, the patient, differently at a certain stage of life or with a specific disease. You are treated as an equal and not talked down to. The provider is kind and thoughtful and treats you with respect.

As my research progressed, I sensed a genuine need for education on the part of both the providers and the patients. Mastering the art of listening and communicating is not a process taught to the general public in schools, and more education is needed in medical schools as well. This type of training would improve every office visit when used and accepted by society in general. The hierarchy paradigm does not work for the majority of patients I interviewed. They want a more equal relationship with their health care providers. I believe this alone would improve our system of health care and create happier patients and providers.

The current system may be unable to accommodate this type of training at present, but it is possible. What is necessary for this to occur is a change of perspective. Patients are people, and they want to be valued and cared for. Providers want to be given the time and environment conducive to treating their patients successfully. Patients and providers are not commodities and strongly resent being treated as such by the health care system. We have all heard the saying "What goes around comes around." It does. When providers give the patients what they need, and when the system gives the providers the time and training to do it, the results can be nothing but positive.

5

THE SKILLED HEALTH CARE PROVIDER

*To be faithful to your instincts and the impulses that carry you in the
direction of the excellence you most desire and value...surely that is to
lead the noble life.*

~GEORGE E. WOODBERRY

M EDICAL EDUCATION IN the United States is considered to be among the
best in the world. When compared to those of many other countries,
the standards of medical care are high, especially related to high-tech advances.
The requirements for entrance to medical schools are high as well. When a
provider graduates from an accredited medical school in this country and is
licensed, most patients expect that the provider is competent. They count on
this. Patients want competency and honesty. They realize that as times change
and new scientific discoveries are made, it is necessary for their providers to

continually educate themselves to stay current. Some patients do research themselves, but others are dependent on providers to keep them up to date.

However, there is a remarkable amount of science that is not embraced by the majority of physicians. The medical school curriculum's main focuses are biology, chemistry, and disease. However, there is a growing number of providers who realize their patients' interests in complementary treatments outside of the standard of care. The medical profession's response is that it is waiting for the proof through research. Much of the science exists but is unknown to the vast majority of allopathic physicians. Altering the standard of care is a complicated process. I will address that further in the chapter dealing with treatment options.

A physician of over thirty years stated that physicians in general are not really trained for multi-illness: "Sometimes we convince ourselves that when patients have multiple problems, they are due to psychological problems, so it is not our fault when they don't get better. The patients most difficult to treat are often the most poorly treated on the emotional level." This affirms the need for providers to see the person as more than a disease, but a person with unique experiences.

In my own personal experience, conventional medical doctors do not have time to understand my complicated medical history. In addition, it is a serious task to find a good primary care physician who is taking new patients. I finally found one who is a doctor of osteopathy. She took thirty minutes to listen to my medical issues but referred to my beliefs and unconventional self-care as idiosyncrasies. I was just grateful that she did not suggest that I stop them. When the doctor received my exemplary lab results, she told me to continue doing whatever I was doing. What I am doing is in no way conventional and stems from my own motivation to learn as much as I can about how to maintain good health. Most patients are not as motivated as I am and need more support.

In the current health care system, there is a real lack of primary care doctors. These are the docs whose job it is to see the whole picture—the patient's mind, emotions, and lifestyle, as well as the physical signs of illness. These work together and affect each other. Most patients are keenly aware of this and feel cheated when they are treated as the disease or the illness with little concern for who they are. In some cases, a caring nurse, assistant, or coach may be able to provide some support, but it then becomes essential for the health care provider to work with others as a team to acquire the whole picture of the patient's condition.

Common sense is underrated. Science and double-blind studies are useful and necessary, but so is common sense. Many great experiences that patients have are specifically because their providers used common sense to treat them. They used less invasive methods of treatment or just gave the issues some time before taking action. The body has a magnificent ability to heal itself when given the chance. Physicians stated that with experience comes the ability to make wise decisions regarding when to use common-sense measures and postpone treatment.

In general, patients appreciate primary care doctors who make appropriate referrals to specialists and know when to refer. Some people, however, have had the experience of being sent to many different specialists, making it almost impossible for any of those providers to see the whole picture. Some patients complained that they were misdiagnosed for years. Larry (not his real name) stated, "If I have a serious situation, I would like the provider to give me the time I need. The time needs to match the situation I am in. I had a practitioner misdiagnose me and give me cortisone shots when I did not respond well to the physical therapy. Six months later when my complaints continued, the provider suggested more cortisone without having ordered an MRI. Over time, when I knew something was still wrong, I did not go back to the primary care doctor but to a sports medicine doctor. I was told that I did not have a sprain but a torn tendon." Larry feels that he knows his body and that had he been more forthright in his communication with the primary care physician or had the provider asked for Larry's input, he would have had an MRI before drug treatment and would have healed much sooner.

Another story of a disappointed patient and poor communication came from a woman named June (not her real name). June had a long history of high cholesterol and nasty side effects from taking numerous statin drugs—debilitating pain. She did not want to take another one. Her cholesterol was close to normal, and she was on a stricter diet now. She explained all of this in detail to her new physician on her second appointment with him. The physician dismissed what June said and stated that he wanted her cholesterol checked again and that if June was pain free (from statin side effects) he would try her on a different drug, Prevastatin. June knew it was just a different statin and asked the physician why he thought that one would help her. His answer was, "'Cause I said so." June told me, "I don't think he heard a word I said." She will not be returning to that physician for care.

The combination of time limitations and providers diagnosing medical issues without input from patients can create an environment ripe for errors in diagnosis and treatment.

To reiterate, providers who are open to knowing their patients will find that patients' input increases their ability to provide the best treatment. No two patients are the same. Yes, there are similarities, and the basic science of the body doesn't change considerably, but an individual's response to life and treatment can be very different: "All human beings are not the same. He [the provider] needs to know the personality of the patient so that he might know what the diagnosis means coming from you." This is common sense, but it requires practice and time to become skilled in this area.

A patient describes his perspective: "In the competition to lower cost, what is lost is the ability to take time to see the whole picture. I see this as a project manager working with an architectural plan that has cut costs. In lessening the cost for the customer, something is lost. It is like providing the standard of care [for patients], instead of creating something that works specifically for this project. Every project is different." And every person is different.

Patients also want honesty in their relationships with their providers. "I don't know the answer to that question, but I will look into it" is a statement that most patients would like to hear occasionally from providers of care. In the experiences of nearly all the patients I interviewed, this is rare.

Why? Perhaps time limitation is an issue. In addition, little room is made for the admission of limitations in knowledge within a system where medical professionals have been raised to high social status and, in some cases, have a godlike image projected onto them. Many providers find it difficult to admit that they don't have all the answers. But they do not. No one could. With all the knowledge and incredible tools health care providers have, there is an equal amount of knowledge they do not have. The body is extremely complex, and there continues to be much we do not know.

Another area of concern when you are on the receiving end of care is that of medication. In the high-tech world we live in, information overload is common. On the Internet, television, and billboards, drugs and the promise of instant healing are prolific. Television ads tout beautiful, happy people saved from their despondent and miserable lives by the wonder drug of the moment. Anxiety and stress abounds, and people sometimes see these ads as the answers to all their problems. It behooves the provider to resist the easy way out and instead offer other means of healing.

Patients want to get well, and they want options: "I want choices presented. If I have a problem, I don't just want a drug." Although some overwhelmed patients state they will initially ask for medication, when further questioned, these same people would prefer options and encouragement. Often, people depend on providers of care to set limits.

Being the receiver of care exposes a person to a variety of different experiences in the office and hospital setting. Most interviewees complained that the waiting time in a provider's office was too long. They see this as a lack of respect for their time and as evidence of poor business skills.

In emergency rooms, doctors and staff might do well to learn how to quickly differentiate between emergencies and nonemergencies without making people wait for two to five hours. That is inhumane. I have had that experience with a loved one, and it is so unpleasant and very difficult when the patient is already suffering. Urgent-care establishments have solved this problem to a point, but emergency rooms continue to be unreliable in offering people respect and courtesy.

People want providers to have a good business sense and to be able to provide patients with a clean and organized office space and efficient staff with a calming and welcoming attitude. They don't want to be moved from one space in the office to another like sheep being herded. A provider of care who understands what a healing environment is and makes that available to his or her patients adds a level of healing that is deeply appreciated and welcomed. It may take some research and a caring attitude, but it is the provider's responsibility to offer that to his or her patients.

The environment of stress seems to be the norm for many health care providers' offices today. Making a patient wait for a long time is stressful and makes a person feel like just a number. It is disconcerting to wait forty-five minutes to an hour to see a practitioner. In addition, it is stressful for the provider when he or she has a waiting room full of people who need to be seen. Many patients described feeling rushed and unable to take the time they need to deal with their issues. Time management is a stress-management technique, and many patients truly appreciate a provider who handles appointments well. That skill reduces stress for both patients and practitioners.

In the Stanford studies on stress, Luskin and Pelletier affirmed that working under stress makes a person less productive. To work in a system that diminishes well-being in both providers' and patients' lives produces an additional amount of stress beyond what the illness itself causes. When energy that is expended to handle stress is used instead to learn what would work better, the medical system will be greatly enhanced, and the improved management skills will benefit both the providers and their patients. As a patient myself, I appreciate a provider who knows his or her limitations and schedules appointments appropriately, even when that means seeing less patients that day.

As long as we continue with business as usual, the possibility of producing empathetic and competent providers is unlikely. The main purpose—to provide good health care to human beings—is being overlooked in many office and medical-education settings. Nearly every person I interviewed mentioned the word *caring* as part of the provider skill set they desired. Most of the physicians and providers of care that I interviewed stated that within the confines of the current health care system in the United States, they are unable to give the kind of care that their patients need. And the patients are not satisfied either. In many ways, they feel mistreated.

In a system with out-of-control health care costs and nearly epidemic chronic diseases, a new direction is necessary. The combination of overworked physicians and health care providers, stressed-out staff, and undervalued patients is a recipe for failure. How can a provider of health care give good care to his or her patients when he or she is not taking care of him or herself? Something will be lost in the process. The best teachers/mentors in the world are those who walk their talk. Patients know when their providers practice what they preach.

This shift in focus can be taught in every institution of higher education that pertains to health care. Patient-centered care is being touted as a great idea whose time has come—the future of medicine—but actions speak louder than words. And every patient who walks into a practitioner's space or hospital is keenly aware of it: "Truth, honesty, integrity, and compassion need to come back to the health care system."

6

PARTNERSHIP

Alone we can do so little; together we can do so much.

~HELEN KELLER

I HAD AN interesting conversation with a man who only recently had the experience of needing to obtain medical care on a regular basis. He said, "The existing view is that they [the patients] give control to the doctor—that puts all the responsibility on the system or doctor. Ideally, medical care would be where the doctor explains what he or she found and talks about various options that may exist and the possibilities there are for healing with each. Based on that, I would make a decision."

In the input I received from some physicians, they don't like for patients to tell them what they want to do to maintain good health. I understand how patients wanting to take the lead on treatment could occasionally be problematic for the provider. But in interviewing patient after patient, listening to them talk about their experiences in health care, I saw a pattern arise. Many people want to be part of the decision-making process. They want to be partners in their health care decisions.

They want to be able to question the providers and express their thoughts about the treatments. It can also encourage compliance when patients are considered in creating treatment plans. It is taking ownership of their individual plans. Many people are more willing to take responsibility for their parts of the plans when they have a say in them. I know this from experience with my own clients.

One female patient stated, "I want to participate in my health care. I will drop a doctor if he does not give me good care and I will shop for another one. I will try the care of my physician, but do not see him as God. I will stop treatment if I think it is hurting me. I will speak up to my doctor and want a doctor who respects my opinion." She has had numerous experiences in the health care system and knows her way around. Her opinion is not rare, however. I heard similar feelings from the majority of people I spoke with. They want to be part of the equation. Here are some related comments:

Regarding partnership, the following quotes from both patients and providers speak for themselves.

"I want to be part of the decision-making process and want someone open to listening to what I desire."

"I need to do my homework and be a responsible patient. I want to work in partnership with my doctor."

"I want to be a partner in my care and always be informed. I know my body and I take responsibility for it. Patients need to be good historians."

"I want to be a partner in the care...I want my opinion valued. I want them to listen to me and value what I say. I want someone open to all of that. It's my body. You would never know it from my experiences."

"If I did not speak up and take care of my body, I would be a victim of any negative consequences that occurred because of my lack of participation. I want to be a partner in my care...I know my body and I take responsibility for it."

"I want my patients to be real partners in this process. We are going to try and come up with a plan that we think will fit them the best. To make that work, I want them to participate and do the plan as best as they can, but also giving me feedback so that we can actually try and find out what really works for them and what does not...I do want patients to partner with me. They are in charge of their health, and I want them to take responsibility for their health."

"Patients, those more involved, they follow directions."

"Some of my patients like that I have a reason for what I am doing and can explain it. I feel like it is their body. They want a partner for increased health and pain relief."

"Patients need a medical cocaptain."

These are just a few of the comments valuing partnership between patients and their providers. There were many more.

In *Merriam-Webster*, one definition that fits the provider-patient partnership is described as "a relationship resembling a legal partnership and usually involving close cooperation between two parties having specified and joint rights and responsibilities." The patients I spoke with want to be understood for who they are and want providers to respect their beliefs when important decisions are being made for their treatment. A good rapport with the provider and participation in their own care is essential for patients.

More than half the people I interviewed mentioned integrated care. They want treatment to reflect who they are as whole people, what affects their well-being, and what works well in their individual lives—that includes personal life issues. Although this may not be covered in medical schools in detail, as I've mentioned before, it is a component of care that can make the difference between positive and negative outcomes. "[I want to see] more mandatory education in medical schools in this area," stated a patient who takes responsibility for her own health. A nurse stated that she thinks that "quick, unconcerned care is detrimental to a patient's overall health."

On the whole, those patients who take responsibility for their health and want to partner with their providers reported health care experiences that were more positive with better health outcomes. They do not feel like victims, do not see the providers as God figures, are knowledgeable, speak up for themselves, and demand respect from their providers. They want to be part of the process and make it known to their practitioners. I did not have the opportunity to interview a large number of conventional physicians, but those I did speak to have time-constraint issues with this type of relationship. I heard the time-constraints issue repeated over and over in all my interviews with both providers and patients.

Coordination of care is considered to be of great importance according to most people I interviewed. There were complaints of doctors not passing on medication information or providing incorrect information, paperwork and test results not being shared with other providers caring for the patient, and errors being made due to the lack of good communication. Electronic medical records are becoming more common and may handle some of these issues; however, the personal touch is repeatedly stated as essential to most patients and many providers of care.

I know from my experience in case management some years ago that good plans for people and their families always involved the team approach. Different aspects of the team had different information and different ways of advocating for the individuals and their families. They all had something to add to the true picture of how to improve the lives of the people they served. One team member was not necessarily more important than another. Everyone made a contribution—most importantly, the individual being served.

What is being conveyed here is that being a skilled team player is highly desirable in health care today. Many voices and points of view are needed to see the whole picture of a patient's illness and to acquire the best results in health care. There is no one right voice. However, this is not the common experience of most patients today. Although some people are naturally more skilled in this area, for most it requires education and practice to improve the common provider-patient relationship.

An RN I interviewed feels very strongly about the provider of care adequately informing patients of "medical information or information of studies that have been done that they are aware of that I am not. I want someone who keeps up with current scientific information and literature." She also desires someone who can help solve her problems and who can help her to maintain her health for her age. She admires a provider who can admit when he or she does not know the answer and "who is sincere, honest, and forthright."

It is important to note that patients who take responsibility for their care and feel they are partners in their care arrive at providers' offices with lists of questions, complaints, and other pertinent information. Common sense dictates that when a patient is clear and concise, the provider has the information necessary to make a more complete and accurate decision about care. The patient who feels that he or she is in partnership with the provider is the same patient who arrives at a visit with an attitude of openness to the provider's treatment plan.

About one-third of the people I interviewed were interested in working in partnership with a practitioner who was open to more natural, complementary methods of treatment. They wanted to feel free to mention these methods and discuss possibilities. This can be part of the relationship when the provider is adequately educated on the scientific basis for these complementary methods of treatment. Most of the providers I spoke with who are educated in this realm learned independently of their formal medical training.

Part of the oath physicians take is to do no harm. Learning to use less invasive techniques before turning to a barrage of medications, tests, and procedures can be cost effective and have very good outcomes.

A male patient living in a more progressive state who originally came from a more conservative one said that he has noticed that the providers where he lives now are more open to going outside of the realm of "standard of care" and taking a more commonsense approach. He said, "There is more openness out here." This patient is very involved in his care and works together with his health care providers when determining the correct treatment plan.

An element of care that is often overlooked is one of spirituality and community. One interviewee stated, "Belief in a higher power that I can connect with to support me in trying times is also part of good health." His viewpoint is not uncommon and is supported by research. Although this was not a common thread in my interviews, the patients who used this type of support were more inclined to take responsibility for their health and make necessary changes when appropriate.

There is a great deal of evidence that patients who have a supportive belief system or community in place have better medical outcomes. Support from a higher power, family, friends, or a community is essential to the emotional needs of people, especially when an individual is ill or facing a serious disease. It behooves practitioners to embrace and encourage this kind of support in caring for their patients, asking each patient about his or her personal support system.

That is where listening and good communication can be invaluable. Some people I spoke with have little support, and that greatly decreased their abilities to follow treatment plans and maintain hope during their illnesses. The provider of care needs to acknowledge this when working with his or her patients.

I have a physician who I can talk to about my spirituality and the important people in my life; it is very helpful to be able to bring that into the doctor's office. It is essential to my life and to my well-being, as it is to many of the patients I spoke with. However, this is not a subject that most providers readily discuss with patients. Yet encouraging patients to have a good support system (whatever that is for them) is invaluable in creating good health outcomes. Because my physician really knows who I am and wants to work together with me on my health issues, I immediately feel comfortable when I sit down in his office; I feel supported as a whole person. I am not a disease or an illness; I am me and need to be a partner in my healing process.

Another tool to utilize a patient's strengths is to note when a patient is feeling helpless or hopeless. This emotional state is often associated with victimhood, lack of motivation, and the inability to make changes. Patients or clients who feel they can't change their circumstances and have no power over them are discouraged and unable to move forward. This lack of motivation can keep patients stuck and unable to follow treatment plans.

Some patients told me that a good rapport with a provider who respects them and encourages them also empowers them, gives them hope, and increases their motivation. They want a provider who knows them and believes they have some control over their health outcomes. One patient told me she feels that many practitioners she has had experience with in this country don't believe patients will follow their treatment plans. Some providers of care I interviewed have expressed that very sentiment. This is another valid reason to listen and communicate as partners in health care. Respecting the patient as an equal partner creates an environment where patients are more likely to take action for better health. That is something we would all like to see.

7

WHAT ARE THE OPTIONS?

We are our choices.

~Jean-Paul Sartre

AMERICANS LOVE CHOICES. Walk into a grocery store, and you are faced with more than forty-five thousand different items to choose from. We love shopping malls and farmer's markets, cultural festivals, online shopping, and forty different flavors of ice cream. It is the status quo, and we would be lost without it.

There is a dark side to too many choices. Like anything else, there is a limit to the amount of choices that provide optimal satisfaction. Too many choices and you can feel overwhelmed, and it can cause additional stress. People love choices, but just the right amount…not too much. Having choices in health care is no different.

The health care field has become very complicated. There are new discoveries, new technologies, and new rules and regulations and procedures. Health care providers do their best in the United States to keep up, but there are forces other than what we see when we walk into a medical office or facility that are strongly affecting our customary care. There are insurance companies, pharmaceutical companies, medical-equipment companies, and corporate pressures that also mold our experiences in any health care environment.

Most of the people I spoke with struggle with the immensity of the system, but when a patient is face-to-face with the health care staff, they are not concerned with that—they just want respect and good care. The majority of patients know the pressures out there. They feel it the moment they enter the space. They want to feel comfortable and calm, and they resent it when they have to wait too long and feel like a number.

As one male patient said, "The process is brutal, impersonal, and tends to make me feel like a piece of meat, moved from place to place, [the doctor] spending only a few minutes with me, the patient, and then he or she goes onto the next patient." In addition, nearly every patient I spoke to wants to wait only about fifteen minutes to see a very busy provider, and for their favorite provider, who gives them the time they need, no longer than thirty minutes. Anything else is unacceptable to them. This, of course, is not the norm.

A holistic physician held that "the regular health care system does not allow for much time, and it usually takes a certain amount of time for people to tell any practitioner what is really on their mind. In standard practice, they are thinking about three things at once and are thinking about how to bring the visit to a conclusion about three minutes after the visit has started."

This type of visit was the common complaint of almost every patient I spoke with. It is also a good reason for a caring provider to work outside of the conventional system. Larger and larger numbers of providers are making that choice and creating their own private practices, where they can provide their patients with the individualized care they require. Although much of the treatment they will provide is covered by insurance, some is not.

There is a sense among health care recipients that "the institutions appear to be too big to care." More time per patient is needed to give good care, and currently that is the exception. One man stated that he wants the time he spends with his doctor to match the medical complaints. If it is serious, he wants more time. That is seldom the option given him. He is willing to make it a short visit if his complaint is minor but feels slighted when he needs to discuss something and the time to do that is not available. This choice is not given to patients as a whole. The system puts people in a box and treats them in a similar manner. As I have said before, patients want to be treated as individuals with their own sets of circumstances, not as bodies with working parts that can break down.

Patients who are seen in a private practice and not a huge conglomerate generally have more time to be cared for. Holistic doctors and other nonconventional practitioners see the need for this and do well in accommodating their patients. Patients greatly appreciate the personalized care. However, this is generally done outside of the corporate domain and is not possible for those patients who have financial constraints.

People generally would like to have the option to choose this type of care, but insurance companies place limitations on the practitioners. Some of these professionals forego the constraints, take a loss, and give their patients the care they deserve. These practitioners provide many different choices to their patients and in my experience give the kind of care that we received thirty years ago.

I questioned a physician about how we as a society can get back to the family-doctor type situation, and she told me she didn't know how to get back to a more caring system. There are volumes of information on different options for medical care, but according to those practitioners outside the conventional system, their kind of care is possible only when they work independently. Some people have experienced the old-fashioned kind of care in the larger facilities, but it is not common, and when patients come across it, it is a breath of fresh air.

Another problem with limited choices is when people covered by insurance companies have to change providers because their provider left the insurance company they are with: "Often, the plan changes, and doctors leave the plan. This causes inconsistency in care." Clearly, our choices as patients are limited. It takes time for a patient-practitioner relationship to develop to a point where it is beneficial to patient care. More value needs to be placed on continuity of care. It will be more efficient, will benefit the system financially, and will make practitioners happy as well.

Options, with regards to the kind of care received, are a concern to many of the patients I interviewed. Most claim they do not want the most invasive treatment first, and they don't want a lot of X-rays and other expensive tests. They prefer a provider who, through his or her knowledge of medicine, the patient, and the situation, as well as through his or her intuition, will make an educated guess and give the situation more time prior to more invasive treatment and drugs. Many people prefer the opportunity to change their lifestyles and diets before going on to other treatments.

In patient interviews, the desire for these options was repeated over and over again. But because of the standard of care being the go-to answer for most providers, providing options for care is not often the case. The standard of care is also the type of care that conventionally trained providers are most comfortable with. In fact, their licenses can be in jeopardy in some situations if they do not follow the standard. This keeps options at bay. It is believed to be safest overall for the patient, but it may not be the most effective way to treat an individual and may cause a patient's health to deteriorate if that care is not ideal for him or her.

The argument for utilizing complementary-medicine practitioners is that their care can and does often save patients time when the illness is resolved and money when they don't have to have expensive tests or drugs. It makes sense to try less invasive, safer treatments first before sending patients to different practitioners, taking tests, or trying drugs. One of the main issues is that many options holistic practitioners provide their patients are not taught in medical school, and thus most patients do not have the opportunity to make these choices in their conventional care.

An educator who had worked extensively in the medical field talked about the need for change in regards to options for treatment. She wants "the health care delivery system to be more integrative and holistic; the holistic embraces Eastern and Western—an integrated health approach to health and healing." She knows of some "leaders in health care who have this mind-set, and this is good news."

Common sense in care needs to be given more value in interactions between patient and provider. That type of care takes time and focus as well as experience. One patient mentioned, "Most providers don't give me much guidance…unless I have something really bad, they tell me very little. They don't give it their attention unless it is a disease." People want some guidance in their everyday lives where choices are made that can affect their health. Encouragement and guidance are values that patients want to see in health care situations. As a wellness coach, I know that discussion and guidance in regards to lifestyle changes can make all the difference in whether or not a patient gets well.

Until conventional medical education begins to embrace the fact that patients want to be seen as more than bodies or diseases and need to be treated as such, much of the care that patients get will be the standard of care. Given that patients want more than just disease management, it behooves practitioners to be more open to options that are safe. It is, however, important to note that the conventional methods of treatment are not perfectly safe—nothing is because any patient can respond differently.

Recently, I have read numerous articles about the dangers of utilizing complementary medicine over the standard of care. The providers who write the articles and refer to holistic practitioners as quacks and some complementary modalities as magic or voodoo show their ignorance when making comments like these. There is science behind many of the modalities used, but the provider must be willing to research and look for it.

I find this constant criticism curious, given that the majority of the population uses this type of care. Although I understand that there is limited understanding of the complementary modalities among conventional providers, it is their responsibility to learn about them. Patients want to use them.

A fraction of the patients I spoke with refuse to try complementary modalities without the approval of their primary care doctors. They follow authority regardless of the situation. This is unfortunate for the patient because as one registered nurse said, "It is sad for people who don't speak up. I always want to be informed and know my options for treatment. People need to be good historians." In addition, often the patient who wants to be taken care of does not always share necessary information with his or her provider, and this can and does cause errors. This patriarchal model of care is slowly disappearing with the older generation as more and more people decide to be active instead of passive in their medical care.

Most patients that I interviewed learn about complementary remedies on their own or are referred by their friends and families. Yoga has now become mainstream, and a good yogi will provide a holistic, healing environment for his or her classes. As this trend continues and patients share their successes with complementary/holistic modalities, more and more patients will request it. In turn, this will encourage conventional providers to learn more about it. There is no alternative for feeling great, and if complementary care does that for patients, they will use it. It is really that simple.

Good nutrition and a balanced lifestyle are essential components of complementary medicine protocol. About a year and a half ago, I attended a nutrition lecture at a very large teaching hospital. Following some questions and answers that he put to the audience, the researcher commented to the mostly nonmedical audience that we answered his questions more accurately than the medical students he teaches. We live in a time when more and more research is confirming that healthy lifestyle and diet are essential for good health. When the public knows more about nutrition than medical students, we have a problem in our medical-school education.

Several of the physicians I spoke with recently stated that the younger medical doctors are showing more interest in complementary treatments. They know it is here to stay and are basically more open to it. The Internet, of course, has played a huge role in patients and providers learning more about different options for health care. More and more websites with credibility are showing up to provide valid information to both patients and providers.

It will be helpful to patients and beneficial to society in general when conventional providers educate themselves on complementary treatments or insist that medical schools offer mandatory course work in this area of expertise. Currently, it is extremely lacking in medical schools, and there is more scientific proof available than most providers are aware of.

Due to this dilemma, many conventional practitioners refuse to consider these options for their patients. One patient stated, "Alternative [complementary] methods are absolutely necessary. Medical schools don't teach them. Look at the whole body, the whole person, spirit and all." Another wants to be offered "a different approach to stopping a disease." Another patient "want[s] doctors to learn more holistic methods and use them in treatment."

The options that patients desire are not yet widely available. A professional woman who works with medical practitioners states, "Change needs to come from all of the key stakeholders. The culture of our system is not yet patient centered. Patients need to become more assertive and take more ownership of their health care. This is a paradigm shift." I concur. Empowering patients will cause substantial positive changes in the way health care is delivered.

8

THE PATIENT'S VIEW ON
HEALTH INSURANCE

We must not allow other people's limited perceptions to define us.

~VIRGINIA SATIR

"INSURANCE IS STILL dictating health care ninety percent of the time," states a discouraged health care provider. From a patient's perspective, that is a bit scary. Why should insurance companies be telling my health care provider what kind of care I should have? One patient phrased it like this: "The health insurance companies need to stay out of the doctor's office. The doctor's office door should say, *The buck stops here*." I wish it were that easy.

A number of providers I interviewed work very hard to give their patients the best care; however, health-insurance companies make that very difficult at times. The providers or experts in their fields know what type of care will improve the patient's health, but their hands are tied when the patient is not financially able to self-pay for the care the insurance company has limited. Insurance companies are trying to keep their costs down and therefore cut care wherever they can. But insurance companies often do not have control over the original cost of care, especially in larger institutions.

In 2013 journalist Steve Brill wrote a comprehensive article for *TIME* magazine addressing the high cost of medical care. The author stated that in a hospital there is a charge master. This is the hospital's internal list that notes the cost for every item used in the hospital. In this list the hospital charges seventy-seven dollars for gauze pads that may cost one dollar in a drugstore. The pharmaceutical companies that sell the drugs to the hospital make a huge profit, and the hospital marks up the price as well. There are no regulations regarding these costs, and the costs are unsustainable.

Because the cost of care often is exorbitant, patients cannot afford to go without insurance. Even with medical insurance and very good plans, the co-pays are high, and people have gone bankrupt after contracting serious illnesses, even losing their homes in the process. For many people, this is not acceptable, especially in such a powerful and wealthy country.

Cancer treatments can be hundreds of thousands of dollars. A physician stated that "the cost of a colonoscopy can be anywhere from $1,000 to $5,000. It is insane." One woman with a broken ankle who had adequate health insurance received a bill for $900 from an emergency room visit. The bill contained "no information, no detail—it looked like they expected me to pay it without question, which is probably what a lot of people do." She obtained a detailed bill only after she called and requested it.

The average person today does not have the financial stability to pay for medical care on their own. Patients I spoke to without health insurance most often did without medical care. In some cases, friends or community members would help them connect to a free source of care when they needed assistance. These people research natural cures they can administer themselves or in very serious cases go to a hospital emergency room. They suffer through the illnesses and often only seek professional care when they have chronic or serious diseases. One patient stated, "People need to be valued. Right now the value of people does not matter [in the health care system]."

Access to health insurance is another serious issue for many patients. Today, those who work part time are usually not offered health-insurance benefits as part of their compensation. Some companies, such as Walmart, have been accused of purposely keeping hours down to avoid paying for health insurance for their employees. Most full-time employees still obtain health-insurance coverage through their employers.

The option of self-pay is unreasonable for those who consider themselves middle class, as well as for those working people who cannot keep up with the cost of living. Medical care is just too expensive. Many times those least able to pay for their insurance are those who are also unable to afford medical care out of their own pockets.

The majority of people who responded to the question of health insurance told me they believed all people should have access to high-quality health care. One individual suggested that the cost of health care needs to be determined by the needs of the individual: "Free for poor people, low cost for middle- and high-income people, subsidized by tax revenue." Others felt that universal health care was the answer to this problem: "I think everyone deserves good care." Of all the patients I spoke with, not one believed people should be denied health care when needed.

Many citizens in our country do not fully understand the health care system, and they don't know what to expect when they are faced with illnesses or diseases. Experiencing an illness can strike terror in the hearts of a family who has no health care insurance and can barely make ends meet. The fear alone adds to their stress and does not provide the environment conducive to healing. Stress is an underlying element in most of the common diseases in the United States.

To put a personal face on living without health care insurance, I will share a personal experience of mine, which suggested to me that those without health insurance get the bare minimum of care, even in emergencies. I was in the ER with a friend who had broken her ankle; she had insurance and got appropriate X-rays and good care. On leaving the facility, we spoke with a man on crutches with his ankle wrapped with gauze and some support. He was complaining vehemently about the inappropriate care he had received because he didn't have insurance. Pointing to his foot, he said, "This is what I get—they told me to follow up with my doctor." He was both frustrated and fatigued. I would expect that this is not an isolated case. There is a great advantage in having health care insurance in situations such as these.

The US health care system preaches prevention and encourages all people to see their doctors regularly, but they are only speaking to those with health insurance. These kinds of visits do not occur among those struggling to pay their bills. Only the wealthy can afford to self-pay for care, and the majority of those who can pay have health insurance.

Another reason to offer health care to all is that those who do not have health care insurance and frequently do not get preventive care ignore physical symptoms of illnesses until they are in crisis and end up in the emergency room of a hospital. "People need to go to the doctors before they are sick, not when they are really sick and need intense medical care. Emergency rooms are not the place for patient care—it is for emergencies," states a concerned RN. Yet there is little recourse for those who cannot afford to pay. In addition, where urgent care centers are not available and public transportation is a patient's only choice, the emergency room is the logical place to go.

A patient recalls, "I am very familiar with having no diagnosis at all. When I did not have any insurance [after college], I did not go to the doctors at all. I tried to take care of it myself or just forget about it. I might try to work on my mental health and hope that I would get better—do common-sense things. I would also pray a lot that it was not really bad." This is the story of many uninsured people.

Millions of people without health care insurance was the issue that brought President Obama to push for the Affordable Care Act (ACA). This act has assisted millions of people who otherwise could not afford health care or health insurance. Preventive care is also encouraged and in some cases required in the ACA. The act affects different people in different ways, but overall it works to balance out the cost in most insurance situations. Some pay more, and some pay less. It does offer insurance to most Americans, and we have all heard the stories of people going bankrupt in this country because of medical-care costs—with and without insurance. However, the ACA does not directly lower the cost of care. This is one of the law's greatest issues.

Health care insurance is very complicated, and all plans are different and can be very confusing for the recipients of care. In some instances, those who self-pay due to being uninsured or because a given treatment is not covered in their plan pay more for the service than if it were covered. For example, if my insurance does not cover a specific treatment, the facility or provider will very likely bill me for the full amount of the treatment, even though had this treatment been covered by my insurance, they would have only received half the fee. How can the health care provider or facility expect an uninsured person to pay the full cost under these circumstances? This inequitable cost of care is contrary to what patients want and deserve and places the burden on those who can least afford it.

As we experience in many aspects of life, health-insurance companies tend to be shortsighted. They focus on short-term gain and neglect to see the whole picture. Medicine often follows this course of action as well. Kill the bacteria, manage the disease and the symptoms. What we fail to see in focusing only on the present issue is what is connected to it—that is, what came before to cause it and what the future consequences are of the current treatment or lack thereof.

Some good examples of this perspective are described by a patient: "Sometimes instead of paying for maintenance chiropractic care, the insurance company denies it, the person continues to injure themselves until it gets worse, and they then need surgery." Obviously, surgery is more invasive, has a more serious effect on the lifestyle of the patient, and generally the cost is much higher. "Another example is acupuncture for headaches—much less expensive than going to a neurologist and having a CT scan. There is no common sense. It is like trying to be in charge rather than empowering us."

Another patient says, "I want alternatives covered by insurance. I think that type of care needs to be covered. Acupuncture, massage therapy for certain ailments, nutritional coaching for many different diseases—it needs to be covered by insurance as an option to standard care." That is the cry of a great number of the patients I interviewed. They are learning about complementary modalities from friends and family, TV, the Internet, and books.

Self-education is a hobby for many people today, with the Internet making information accessible to the masses. Not all information is equal, and most patients know that; they search out reputable sites. One patient stated that although he does not currently use complementary medicine, he would like it covered if it is effective: "We need to break the power of the conventional medical establishment and insurance industry so as to allow alternative modalities to be given a fair chance."

A provider shared with me that although he has no experience with CAM practitioners, he has patients who do, and they have had positive outcomes. But for many conventional providers, positive outcomes are not enough. They want to see the science. In my extensive experience with conventional medicine providers, there is a lack of openness in the community toward any practices that they did not learn conventionally.

I interviewed about ten complementary medical providers, and every one stated that when they reach out to conventional providers to work as a team, they get little to no response. For the most part, the conventional providers are not interested. Ignorance of a modality does not make it quackery, but in many cases with conventional practitioners, if you don't treat as they do, you're using quackery. There is a distinct aloofness and condescending attitude from conventional medicine toward complementary medicine. This must change. Patients demand it. It would behoove conventional providers to be open to modalities that a majority of the population sees as valid. These providers just may be missing something essential to healing.

Furthermore, nonconventional treatments can bring value to a highly scientifically based system. It is not either-or. For example, the placebo effect is 80 percent effective. Evidently, what people believe can have a powerful effect on them. That is a very high success rate by anyone's standards and higher than many conventional treatment success rates. I'm not suggesting that we throw out science; I am only suggesting that we expand our possibilities for healing.

Since 80 percent or more of Americans believe in a higher power and the power that comes with this belief, it is the height of condescension to think that they (conventional medicine providers) have all of the answers and that their answers are the only ones that are valid. In addition, there is science to back up the protective and healing value of belief in a higher power. It is common sense to pay attention to that and encourage that type of support when appropriate.

A registered nurse with many years of experience shared this: "I want a provider who is willing to share information—any kind of medical information or studies that may have been done that they know about that I don't. I want someone who keeps up with current scientific information and literature." She wants a well-rounded health care provider who is open to new information: "I feel there is too much knowledge out there to know all of it about everything, and specialists are necessary. However, they do need to keep up to date with basic general medicine." The medical profession needs to be more open minded and accepting of their peers' findings and studies." This nurse believes that some complementary modalities have value and should be used and covered by insurance as well.

Scientific research is being undertaken by the federal government agency the National Center for Complementary and Alternative Medicine (NCCAM). Although some CAM treatments are integrated into the conventional setting and are widely used by the US public, it is this agency's goal to develop scientific evidence of CAM treatments to evaluate their effectiveness and safety. This is ongoing and will further the integration of CAM into mainstream medicine.

What I have heard from a few conventional medical providers as well as holistic providers is that the up-and-coming conventional providers are very interested in learning more about the complementary modalities and wellness in general. A blog organized by integrative medical practitioners offered the following websites for conventional health care providers who want to educate themselves about complementary modalities and the science behind them.

They are as follows:

The Institute for Functional Medicine: https://www.functionalmedicine.org/

The Center for Mind-Body Medicine: http://cmbm.org/

In addition, the American College for Advancement in Medicine (ACAM) is committed to the education of physicians and health care professionals, especially with respect to the "safe and effective application of integrative medicine"

(American College for Advancement in Medicine 2015). Their website provides a link for patients to search for a physician in this field of medicine.

There is also a nonprofit whose main mission is to study the effects of nutrition and lifestyle on disease. This group, the American Institute for Cancer Research, is scientifically based and provides a constant stream of information to the public. This is a great service and very necessary in this day and age.

The science is there when one looks for it, and more and more science is proving the benefits of complementary modalities every day. It is time for health care insurance companies and the conventional medical community to take a closer look at what CAM has to offer. It will be an integral part of future health care in the United States.

PART THREE

THE PROFESSIONAL'S PERSPECTIVE

9

EXPECTATIONS AND
PATIENT OUTCOMES

*The fundamental problem most patients have is an inability to love
themselves, having been unloved by others during some crucial part of
their lives.*

~BERNIE S. SIEGEL, M.D.

WHEN ASKING HEALTH care providers what their patients need, I received a variety of answers. The most common response was that they need more time with the patients.

One practitioner in particular was very clear on this issue. She has been an acupuncturist for a long time. During that period of time, she realized that there was one thing all of her patients needed: "They need you to listen to them. No one gets time to be heard." She added that before managed care created a system under the business model, there was more time for patients: "Time management is pushing providers and patients to function within this very small box. Patients want to understand what is going on in their bodies, and most of them don't. Some are old school and won't question the doctor, but the doctor does not give them the opportunity to ask the questions. Most doctors don't have time today."

Another provider says that "patients like my slower-paced practice and that I know them and pay attention to their individual needs. I treat them as individuals."

"When I worked with patients," states an experienced holistic physician, "they said that I was the first person who listened to them and took them seriously. I want to be able to help people, to be able to spend enough time with them to help them. That has fallen off in the last decade. Providers want to be able to have autonomy and treat patients the way they think is appropriate."

Primary care physicians (PCPs) are best known for getting to know their patients and generally spend more time with them. A physician who spent many years in a teaching hospital stated that a PCP "needs to be an expert on where and when to refer patients. The key to good health is that you are going to have a partnership with your primary care physician, yet they are not as highly reimbursed as specialists." Given that fact, it is well known that there is a shortage of primary care physicians and that "even as a physician, access control is difficult as well." Many physicians "go into a higher-paid specialty."

A specialist asserts, "The problem with care today—what has been left out—is time with the doctor and patient, rather than relying on labs and medication. If doctors had the time to listen and figure out the problem, they would not need as many tests. Communication, asking questions of the family and the patient gets accurate information. And tests are more expensive than listening."

This same provider shared a wonderful story that was a great lesson for him:

The best lesson that I had was in junior year of medical school on rotation in a community hospital. It was a very rural area with two excellent interns. I didn't have a lot of experience, and I was told, "I'm sending in a twenty-seven-year-old who is seven months pregnant with diabetes." He told me to evaluate her. I told him that she looked fine, and I ordered tests. He said, "You are not at Johns Hopkins or Stanford—you are paid in chickens, fish, etcetera. Take time to think about the diagnosis and then do the tests." This is a huge problem in all aspects of medicine. The insurance companies don't pay for a doctor's time. Doctors are afraid of being sued, but with better communication, more time [with the patient], and better documentation, you would not have as many lawsuits.

Physicians know their patients expect a skilled provider who is knowledgeable and who cares about patients' well-being. That is common knowledge, but in the real world, what does that mean to providers? They want their patients to follow the treatment plan. A physician states, "I expect patients to be willing to work with me to develop a personalized game plan to address their health problems." That "requires adequate time for patient counseling."

When a new patient walks into the office, a provider needs to not only access the medical issues, but to get a sense of the patient's willingness to follow through with prescribed treatment, explain the treatment thoroughly, and give the patient time to ask questions.

From the responses I received from providers, many patients do not ask questions and do not come forward to share apprehension about the treatment plan—whether it is lack of information, fear, or inability to pay for the treatment recommended. A physician stated, "Patients struggle with understanding their diagnosis, understanding the providers' recommendations, affording costly prescription medications, and being too shy to ask questions of the provider or not knowing what to ask."

Patients come for treatment for illnesses under a myriad of circumstances. Some are educated, some are good communicators and have a certain amount of confidence, but many are not. They need to be educated about their illnesses and have clearly written instructions regarding their treatment plans. If there is any question as to whether the patient will follow through—and providers have shared with me that often it is very clear to them that the patient will not follow the treatment plan—the provider must question the patient and find out why. If the provider does not have the time to do this, someone else needs to offer this service. When this does not happen, the patient remains ill or may become sicker, and no one is helped. The provider is frustrated, and the patient is angry and disappointed. That was clear, especially from the patient interviews.

This is a costly way to do business. It costs patients because they do not experience good health. It costs providers because they want patients to get well and care about the outcomes. It costs the insurance companies and their customers more money in reimbursements and increases in the cost of medical insurance. No one wins.

A social worker of twenty-five years communicated about noncompliant patients and the fact that the majority of chronic illnesses are rooted in stress: "If they really don't move forward, I ask them to look within to see why they don't want to move forward—that becomes the symptom. Fear is usually what comes up...I want my patients to get to the root of the illness." She believes that the answer to this dilemma is "asking more questions, getting more information, and not getting stuck on just the symptoms or what you see...If I focus on one part of a trauma, I would miss the overall picture of their lifestyle."

The practitioner goes on to say that "fear of change is the number one reason for not complying with treatment—what my life will look like, what will I have to do, maybe I should let it go, etcetera." One patient stated that he was overwhelmed with all the changes he would have to make because of diabetes. He said, "[I] just couldn't do it." The therapist gave him one tiny change to make—he agreed to that.

What that patient needed was someone to listen to him for about ten minutes and to motivate and coach him about how to get started. That time needs to be reimbursed as a patient service in order to make it happen. It will not happen otherwise, especially in today's health care system. Many people are struggling to keep pace with the frenetic lifestyle that has become the norm today. They must have some support to make changes. A list of dos and don'ts along with a prescription is just not enough.

This service may be provided by the doctor, nurse, health coach, or another trained professional who can get the entire picture of the patient's circumstances, symptoms, and concerns. It would be a service that, when provided by a professional other than a physician, would be much more affordable and would lower health care costs in general.

Educating patients is also extremely valuable, according to a nursing educator. She said that "many people do not take time to learn about their diagnosis. I think patients just take the information from the doctor and don't explore things further to find out some things they can do themselves to help to heal." She sees self-responsibility as an important part of any healing regimen: "Many people don't understand that they have control over their own health."

However, this educator believes that there are many reasons for noncompliance. Some reasons are "financial constraints...cultural differences...cultural remedies may be used and their diet may be different." If providers do not understand the day-to-day lifestyles of their patients, they may not be able to understand the noncompliance. Patients who are self-pay and have no health care insurance may find it impossible to follow any treatment plan given them. These people will fall through the cracks and show up later in emergency rooms with more serious illnesses.

A massage therapist who treats many patients with chronic illnesses knows the importance of having her patients engage in their healing processes: "They must participate in their own healing...science and healing— for it to work the patient must participate." She has also seen what hope and a positive attitude can do for a patient: "Attitude is a big deal in healing. With negative attitudes, they will not progress." When patients are told they have to "live with it," hope diminishes.

In dealing with the stress of illness, patients expressed that they were told to deal with their stress, but then no other support was given them. How do they do that in their circumstances? A patient who said he has a caring doctor stated, "No instruction was given on how to do that, but he [the doctor] suggested that I deal with my emotional and family issues." In a situation like this, it would be helpful for the provider to refer the patient to another trained staff member, to a professional, or to a support group. Emotional issues can rule a person's life—it is important for the provider to be aware of this and give the patient some guidance. It would improve the compliance issues and result in more positive outcomes.

A practitioner who was not sure how to improve outcomes stated, "Some people listen and some people don't." Then he added, "Patients may not comply with treatment because it is poorly explained, too complex, or they do not want to believe what you are diagnosing." All of this suggests that the patient may not understand, may be afraid or may find the treatment too stressful in his or her circumstances.

A therapist asserts that most people come to therapy "so that they are better at coping with their life challenges." It is essential for any health care provider to understand the stressors in a patient's life. These stressors can make the difference between illness and health. As a health coach, I have worked with clients who had too many stressors in their lives to even consider making any changes. These patients need support from a coach or other professional who can walk them through each challenge one at a time.

Additionally, the appearance of health can lead a patient to become complacent and stop treatment. "Sometimes they don't want to get to the root of the problem and just want to fix it enough to tolerate it," states a caring and conscientious chiropractor. She knows that when her patients begin to get relief, it is time for additional support to help keep the patient on track so there is no relapse: "It works better if I am direct. Many times the patient feels they can tolerate their situation and stops treatment." It is also important for patients to have the "right mix of whatever [treatments] they need in place." She knows when to refer patients to another practitioner and will do so if other treatments improve the patients' conditions.

There is a small minority of practitioners who did not want their patients to educate themselves and come in with ideas about their conditions and possible treatments, but many providers welcome the information and listen for pertinent data to quell their patients' fears: "They want to feel that I am taking their concerns seriously and hearing what they are saying."

This specialist knows that his patients "also look for competence and the skill level they need to address their medical issues." He wants his patients to listen carefully to what he says regarding their treatment and then "I want them to tell me if they are not going to try [the treatment]…and why if they are not going to do it. And I want them to ask questions, feel comfortable and not rushed. I want them to be honest with me and not show up a year later with the same complaint."

Change and the introduction of a different lifestyle are generally understood to be serious challenges in patient compliance. It is difficult to make changes, and providers do not generally have the time to coach patients on motivation and an individualized plan that might work for them. An MD states, "People may put off treatment to maintain the same lifestyle. One cancer patient put off cancer treatment to finish the school year." This could have serious consequences if time is an issue—appropriate support from the health care community is needed to be sure the patient understands the cost of his or her procrastination.

It cannot be emphasized enough that health care providers are frustrated by health outcomes and the lack of compliance by their patients. And patients do not want to run from one provider to another trying to find the treatment that will work for them. It is a huge waste of time, money, and energy on the parts of both the providers and the patients.

I worked in a physician's office for a year and coached many patients who struggled with making the changes that were necessary to improve their health. Patients had different stories, circumstances, and needs. Molding a plan that will work in an individual's life is time intensive. Patience is a necessary virtue for both patients and providers when lifestyle changes are necessary to improve health outcomes. And in almost all cases, real change is required to live a healthier lifestyle.

10

PROVIDING GOOD
PATIENT CARE

*The Art of healing comes from nature, not from the physician, there-
fore the physician must start from nature, with an open mind.*

~PHILIPUS AUREOLUS PARACELSUS

I HAVE NEVER met a physician, nurse, or other health care professional who did
not want to provide good care to his or her patients. Providers' intentions are
good, yet many patients are not getting the care they want and need. There are
various issues with regards to providing good care: access to care, high cost of
care, standard of care, legal liability, coordination of care, insurance reimbursement, and an integrative education.

Access to care has improved with the Affordable Care Act (ACA); however,
there are still many Americans who do not have insurance, and there are rural
areas without care facilities. Even those with insurance may incur health costs
beyond their ability to pay. We live in a country with tremendous opportunities,

yet we do not provide all of our citizens with the security of health care when they need it. Lack of access creates a segment of society that has very limited options when struggling with illnesses and that increases the cost of care overall when their illnesses progress to diseases and must be addressed.

A thorough investigation of the high cost of health care is not within the purview of this book. However, given the power that medical care facilities hold with no regulations regarding hospital, pharmaceutical, and other health care costs, there is no one to rein in the high cost of care. Medicare does attempt to create competition and lower costs, but the ACA provides little relief in this area. Physicians and other providers have limited power in this arena, unless they own health care facilities themselves.

The insurance companies contribute to this problem: "Patients have little incentive to keep costs down because their insurance company covers things that might be unnecessary at times; that is, tests to ease a patient's mind...As a physician, you have to practice defensive medicine to protect yourself, which means sometimes you have to order expensive tests that are not really necessary." This physician stated, "Just the way Pell grants allow colleges to charge obscene fees, the health care system has become totally bloated and overpriced, not answering to anyone; the cost of care is absurd."

Practitioners who work within the insurance-reimbursement system are limited by what the insurance companies allow. Practitioners who are committed to a certain level of care that is not possible within the parameters of the insurance model sometimes set up their own private practices that are self-pay, but that limits the practice to patients who can pay upfront: "Doctors need to be able to treat the patients the way they see fit. Lots of doctors are dropping out of the system to do better care. And then there are many doctors who do not have their own practices now—they work for hospitals."

Other providers offer more time and care to their patients than insurance companies allow by supplementing their incomes in boutique practices. In this model, private physicians offer more time and individual care and charge each patient a flat amount. Again, the financial burden falls on the patient. I contacted a primary care doctor who uses this model, and he charges about $1,300 per year to see him as much as needed. However, this only benefits the patients who present with diseases that need consistent, regular care. This model does not support the needs of a healthy individual without chronic issues.

High cost is also driven by corporations and insurance: "Big Pharma and insurance industries drive things. Drug advertising places obstacles." People come into a doctor's office insisting they must have the newest drug they saw on television or a medical device they saw advertised. A story shared with me was about the commercials for the Scooter Store. The commercials play often and although "Medicare pays $4,000 for a scooter, these same scooters can be bought directly from the company for less than half the price." I am not aware of how cost is established in the Medicare system, but this determination is irrational and very costly.

Another suggestion presented to cut the high cost of health care is to utilize preventive measures and more natural medicine—that is, dietary changes, supplements, lifestyle changes, and stress management. This allows the patient to use less invasive measures before utilizing medication and invasive treatment: "Using natural medicine is a way to improve health and reduce costs, but in this case it becomes crucial for the patient to do lifestyle changes and take responsibility for their own health."

There is great resistance in conventional medicine to using natural methods. Often, it is because these methods are not included in conventional medical training. For many patients it is easier to take a pill than to change their lifestyles. However, there will always be patients who want the quickest and easiest way to handle illnesses, but it is important for the provider to offer them other options.

The conventional model is disease focused; the natural-medical model focuses on maintaining a healthy mind and body. Conventional medical providers believe they are science based and natural medicine is not. This myth is repeated over and over again, mainly because medical students are not offered mandatory training in these areas in medical school and are not aware of the scientific research in area of complementary/natural medicine. Offering different options to patients allows them to choose what works best in their lives. A health care professional states, "Give the patient all of the information they need to make a good decision for themselves."

A patient will not always follow through on this decision, however. Noncompliance is a major issue in providing good care to patients and results in poor treatment outcomes. Some patients clearly do not want to do what it takes for their health to improve. They return repeatedly to the doctor, not having followed care instructions. This racks up health care costs and is very frustrating for both patients and providers.

Patients may provide various reasons why they cannot put the treatment plans into effect, or they may offer no information at all. When the practitioner takes some time to ask relevant questions, it increases the probability that the patient will comply. A physician in a training hospital noted that "the average patient would take responsibility for their health, but setting goals is important and part of the coaching process. Not all people have the will to comply, and chronic stress is not good for people."

The number of patients who are taking responsibility for their health is increasing. Numerous patients that I spoke to understand the importance of independently working on their own health and are willing to take on the responsibility. "Many are interested, educated, and informed. They want to be well and have a healthy life," states a seasoned health coach in an office where that support is provided.

A physician who trained medical students believes that "coaching is one of the roles of physicians, but the patient needs to be brought into that area and educated and motivated to make choices about how to achieve an optimal state of health. The coach role could be the provider or staff member...the patient must be involved. Dependent patients will not be helped—a good example— lose weight—you can't help a person who is not motivated."

This model for patient care is fully supported by providers who use natural medicine in their practices. They know the necessity of self-responsibility in treating patients, knowing that the outcomes will be better and the cost of care less. Support in this area provides many patients with the motivation to make necessary lifestyle changes that improve their health.

Most doctors and other reimbursed practitioners are not allowed time for coaching. This makes a reasonable case for reimbursing health coaching as part of a patient's overall treatment plan. We live in a high-stress world, and in many cases a coach can make all the difference in whether a patient's health improves or he or she becomes a noncompliant patient.

Patients present with many different scenarios, and for practitioners to provide good care, they need to use their intuitions and experiences as well as the standard of care. As an allopathic physician states, "I am willing to work with treatments that make the patients more satisfied. I'm into nutrition myself…I'm more open than the average doctor has been. Patients definitely want a health care provider who is personal and caring, as well as competent. They appreciate a doctor, nurse, or other practitioner who will confidently explain their treatment, clearly explain the instructions, and ascertain whether or not the patient understands. This increases the probability that the patient will comply."

"Patients are more compliant when they trust me and I'm clear about the instructions," notes one provider. A nurse states, "They [providers] need to learn how to teach their patients."

It is clear from all of my interviews that every patient has specific needs according to their states of health, lifestyle habits and circumstances, and genetic tendencies. What is universally known but not strongly encouraged within allopathic practices is a focus on the mind-body connection and on how a person's state of mind affects his or her health. Encouraging and supporting a patient from this perspective can be beneficial and improve outcomes.

There is abundant scientific evidence on meditation and good studies on other practices as well. In conventional medicine, a doctor may tell patients to deal with their emotional issues and their job stresses and may mention meditating, undergoing psychotherapy, or taking some time off, but to make a definitive difference in people's lives takes time, resources, and, in most cases, money. Most relaxation and stress-reducing activities are not reimbursed, and many patients cannot afford them. Once learned, meditation is free and can be done anywhere at any time. Using these modalities would in many cases make the difference between disease and good health.

A common thread woven through my research was the need for self-responsibility on the part of the patient. This standard is not universally accepted by both patients and providers. When asked about how to improve patient outcomes, a physician who worked in public health replied,

"Patients who are educated about their health and how best to maintain and protect it [e.g., beyond being compliant with medications, knowledge about nutrition, physical activity, stress management, and rest], [seeing] physicians who have the time and desire to work with patients, a health care system that reimburses for prevention [including adequate time for patient counseling]" would improve patient outcomes.

This same physician made a statement that all physicians and their patients would benefit from: "I have never met a patient who did not want to be well." Doctors' visits can be intimidating for many patients who feel shy, rushed, afraid, and unsupported. Keeping in mind that all people everywhere need support, thinking past the standard treatment can be lifesaving for many patients who are waiting for their provider to ask, "How can I best support you?" or "How are you?"

The limitations of the standard of care can place obstacles in providing the best care to patients. The standard of care is created by a panel of medical experts. These experts collaborate and specify scientifically based treatments for the general population. Accepted standards are necessary in order to provide patients with appropriate treatment. However, what is often referred to as the standard of care is generally shaped by the predominant health care authority.

By law, these standards need to be evidence based and peer reviewed. This system is used in many cases of malpractice to help determine the judgment. However, there is a risk inherent in this system. When the authoritative system creates the standard of care, it may show bias toward its preferred options for care. Self-promotion is a danger and may exclude reasonable choices that can help patients. Ideally, all schools of thought should be included in the standard of care. A holistic physician stated that it would help if the expert panel creating the standards included those who worked in natural or complementary medicine. It would create a more balanced view for treatment. However, this is not the case. Currently, all schools of thought are not included. It has taken many, many years for acupuncture and chiropractic to be embraced by conventional medicine, in spite of the scientific evidence that they work. And there are numerous studies for many other natural modalities.

Of the conventional doctors I interviewed, one had knowledge of some natural medicine and the science behind it. The physician acknowledged that she is the exception in mainstream medicine. Personally, I have known very few conventional providers of care who were knowledgeable about CAM. Conventional medical education does not mandate that these scientifically based modalities are taught. It is a great disservice to health care providers who may very well utilize these treatments when appropriate for their patients. We must not allow a closed system to impede the progress in health care. Patients need all reasonable options offered them.

A holistic physician noted that he believes the conventional medical community "perhaps should not stifle innovation. On the other hand, those things in the gray area need to be approached carefully." That is where it becomes imperative for conventional medicine to take a good, hard look at the studies that are available for natural medicine. In the health care crisis today, we need all the options on the table. We must not suppress care that is capable of helping patients. This is a moral decision. Many Americans are very sick and getting sicker. Rather than block innovation and consider it as "alternative," whenever possible, it would be wise to integrate CAM and embrace it for the common good.

As mentioned earlier, more than half of the population in the United States uses some form of complementary medicine. Conventional medicine is lagging behind, and both practitioners and patients are suffering because of it. A physician said, "Doctors need more education in natural medicine. We need more patient participation. Doctors should be the teacher and the guide. Health coaches should be in offices to motivate the patients to follow the treatment plan given them. Every medical doctor needs to know how to provide nutritional therapy."

Using complementary/natural medicine could reduce the use of medications, the customary use of which many patients voiced as a major concern. Although some people want a quick fix and want medication, most patients I spoke with would rather have the option of using less invasive treatments prior to taking medications and undergoing other tests and procedures.

Nearly all the patients I interviewed spoke about their frustration with conventional medicine, where there is minimal access to natural methods of treatment, as well as a lack of accurate knowledge about these modalities: "I want my doctor to provide me with different options and not treat me like everyone else." This patient added, "I feel frustrated. I want more information on the condition and options for treatment." Another patient said, "I want my provider to be flexible and open to natural treatments—a mixture of medical and natural is optimal. It seems more and more of them are beginning to understand that, but more often nurses."

Most health care practitioners want to provide the best care for their patients. A physician and public health provider stated, "I see the shift in traditional [conventional] medicine as positive. I still think there is a large core of allopathic physicians who are not ready to embrace holistic practices until they see a specific scientific study that is randomized and controlled. These studies need to be duplicated and there needs to be a consensus on guidelines; we tend to go with the standard of care." She is a believer in the value of integrated medicine, utilizing safe, natural methods as well as conventional treatment when appropriate.

I foresee a time when allopathic and holistic providers will openly communicate with one another. However, nearly all of the holistic providers I interviewed reported that conventional health care providers are hesitant or unwilling to coordinate care for a mutual patient. It was pointed out to me that the allopathic provider does not openly state that however, this unwillingness may manifest in unanswered phone calls or unreturned requests for information or collaboration. On the other hand, conventional medical doctors commented that they had negligible experience with holistic practitioners and that they were unaware of scientific studies that supported natural medicine.

Complementary health care providers are not yet embraced by conventional providers as part of a team who work together to help their patients heal. With more and more patients demanding other treatment options such as CAM, this must change. Education on complementary modalities is needed. More than one physician I interviewed stated that millennial medical students are showing more interest in complementary modalities than their former colleagues. The transition has begun.

11

SYSTEMIC CHANGES

*The world as we have created it is a process of our thinking. It cannot
be changed without changing our thinking.*

~ALBERT EINSTEIN

A SYSTEM THAT puts profits or power before patients will never create a healing environment. It is not possible. How can those in health care provide the best care for their patients when there are time restraints and insurance issues that prohibit them from deeply listening to the patients, gathering essential data to know the whole person, and creating a trusting and caring environment? This is what patients and most practitioners want. "Look at the whole body, the whole person, spirit and all," asserts a patient. Each life is valuable, both to those giving care and those receiving it. When that is the prevailing force in a system, it enables the healer and the patient to bring their best to any situation or illness.

In the current system, there are many very large corporations steering the direction of health care. In some instances this might create new innovations, but for improvement in quality of care for each individual patient, something is lost. As many of the patients I interviewed stated over and over, they feel a lack of personal value in a system that is preoccupied with money and state-of-the-art care. Many feel dehumanized and describe themselves as being treated as a commodity in a system going awry.

The medical-insurance system of care too often puts power into the hands of laypersons. As I have reiterated in this book, patients complain they are not getting the best care under this system. They experience poor treatment from misdiagnosis, delays in treatment due to financial constraints, or lack of insurance. Many patients do not show up at a doctor's office or other provider until the illness or disease has worsened to the point of absolute necessity. Most patients feel unheard, disrespected, and disillusioned regarding the health care system in this country.

It is confusing and disappointing to many patients and to many providers that one of the greatest, most powerful countries on the planet has less-than-exemplary care to offer. Media and those in power, including government agencies, treat the system as infallible and as the ultimate authority, while many laypeople know that is not the case. Unfortunately, this knowledge has been learned the hard way—through experience.

While it is true that we have the greatest capacity for the best medical care on the planet and innovative new treatments are most likely the best, the day-to-day treatment that affects most Americans is unacceptable in various ways, according to most of the patients I interviewed. While those with the power and money argue on what is right and wrong treatment or, even worse, ignore the basic needs of patients in the name of profits, people are struggling with illnesses and diseases that can be prevented. This is morally unacceptable.

The United States touts superiority…what is wrong with this picture?

In considering hospital care, it is far different now from thirty years ago. Furthermore, the nurses I interviewed confirmed the persistent push to do more and more on their shifts, often to stay late to complete paperwork. The nurses felt unable to provide the compassion and care they wanted to give their patients—they do not have time. In addition, the families of patients voiced concern over the fact that their loved ones must have advocates present to get the best care. High productivity is a priority, and there is too much work to be done by the overworked staff.

From a personal perspective, I worked in a major hospital in the 1990s for six years. I know the kind of schedule that the new interns and residents kept even then, and from the reports I am getting from professionals, it is no better or even worse today. It was brutal. Interns and residents experienced huge amounts of stress and were overworked and chronically fatigued. In this strained state, these MDs were taking care of patients and making serious medical decisions. If patients were aware of this, would they choose to have the physicians care for them?

Patients want an educated, competent, alert, and caring practitioner to treat them. The culture within which overwork and stress are seen as badges of honor is not positive or conducive to healing. We pass on what we know. Providers of care need to be educated in the same fashion that they are expected to give care—with competence, compassion, and understanding.

Ralph Waldo Emerson wrote, "Your actions speak so loudly that I cannot hear what you are saying." When a provider who is experiencing stress approaches a patient to treat him or her, the patient feels this stress, no matter what the doctor, nurse, or health care provider says to him or her. The presence of who they are overshadows their words.

Many patients told me they know when their provider is in a hurry, not present to them, or distracted. Human beings have evolved this way for good reason—to protect ourselves from those who might hurt us. Our brains are extremely good at reading a person's face for clues about his or her intentions. Everyone has experienced the discomfort of walking into a room where the tension can be cut with a knife.

It is uncommon to be able to be calm and cool and energetic when we are exhausted and stressed out. Some people are able to do that, and there are times when we all must reach beyond our normal capacities for higher ground. But to have to repeat that on a daily basis is impossible. Often, that is what we are asking of our medical professionals in the current system of health care.

A professional trainer, speaker, and consultant who works with health care providers believes that "the system in this country is broken." She observes a system in transition and believes that "patients will need education and training to help them embrace the new paradigm of patient-centered care." She notes various issues delaying the shift in perception, such as "the cultural assumptions, underlying beliefs, and values about health care delivery."

"What people expect, believe, and value, in some cases, has not shifted with the times. The average person does not have the advantage of having the education and knowledge about how to move through the system successfully. To say 'I'm responsible for my health' is a paradigm shift. Educating the public, helping the public unlearn and relearn a new approach to health care" is required.

Health coaches understand how difficult it is for individuals who have been dependent on the system to take responsibility for the poor individual choices they make that affect their health. Incremental steps are necessary to move a person through lifestyle changes. This is not within the purview of conventional medical practice or within the time limitations of providers. However, among most holistic practitioners, this concept is understood on a very deep level. Furthermore, it would improve patient outcomes tremendously.

For a great many people, life is very stressful, and making serious changes in lifestyle is literally impossible. People need to change from the inside out; they do not change because their doctor or other provider tells them to. They must be motivated by internal pressure, not external. Coaching is a very specific skill that takes excellent training, compassion, and self-knowledge. A good coach is able to facilitate the healing process that the health care provider and the patient desire.

The results of health coaching are being studied currently, and the preliminary results are very positive. There is enthusiasm within the coaching community that within the next decade, coaching will be integrated into the system. In fact, a recent report from a coaching-training corporation notes that by the end of 2015, the standards for health coaches should be completed. It will take another couple of years to create a testing system for certification. That is a game changer.

The consultant/speaker I referred to earlier has spent a considerable amount of time with medical professionals. Having a great deal of experience in the system, this professional is very grateful for the medical resources in the United

States. She readily has access to health care. However, she points out that there are those who do not have access or cannot afford care, "especially the poor and marginalized populations. Quality of care, cost effectiveness, and accessibility is optimal."

She also sees a great need for "more holistic care—the whole body, the whole system, the whole person—an integrated and coordinated approach. Improvement is needed in the area of collaboration across modalities." She states, "The health care delivery system needs to be more integrative and holistic. The medical system is still working in silos; the holistic embraces Eastern and Western, which is an integrative health approach to health and healing. There are some healers in health care who have this mind-set. This is good news."

Health care insurance is an integral part of our health care system. Yet the United States is the only major industrialized nation without universal health care for all. We have Medicare for those sixty-five and older, but maintaining health remains elusive to many people without medical insurance or the financial means to pay for their health care. Medical insurance and adequate health care has become a political football, which makes it very difficult for the citizenry to get the real facts about the current health care system in this county. Politically, there is a spin put on every fact; this causes a great deal of confusion.

Within the last couple of years the ACA, also referred to as Obamacare, has come into effect with great resistance from some politicians. This new program has been beneficial for millions of Americans, yet there is so much misinformation and demonizing of this program, it is nearly impossible to understand. In a nutshell this act has provided health care coverage for more people, added more health care benefits, guaranteed the ability to purchase insurance with or without preexisting conditions, included ten categories of essential benefits to be provided by companies, and overall has had a positive effect on premiums thus far. The subsidies for coverage vary and, similar to car or homeowners' insurance, shift the cost to others.

The cost of health care is not greatly affected by this new law, and time will tell if there are major changes in this area. A physician stated, "If insurance does not pay well, the extreme cost of care drives people away from getting care. In places where there is better access to health care in Europe and Australia, the cost of a colonoscopy is $500 [considerably less than the cost in the United States]. If they don't get the care, they end up in the emergency room, which is very expensive. Then they can't pay their bills." He adds, "Of course it is up to the insurance company what they will and will not pay for; it gets into politics—for example, birth control in Catholic institutions and certain age-group restrictions."

The provider also sees legal liability as an important issue that physicians encounter. He asserts that "legal liability makes doctors do more tests to avoid issues. Specialty doctors make a lot more money, and it limits those who go into primary care, which is very much needed to give the patient good overall care." Moreover, he says, "I have to be careful to not do stuff too far out of the mainstream. Otherwise, I am judged as not providing standard of care. They would say I was practicing bad medicine even without any patient complaints—even if I was responding to a patient's preference. Some of that is good, but on the other hand, it does discourage doing anything too far outside of the norm."

He sees a possible solution: "I would like to see on the medical board a broader representation so that there are other points of view from someone other than conventional MDs. It might be good to have some form of complementary practitioner sitting on the medical board—a naturopath, acupuncturist or even a knowledgeable citizen trying to help provide diversity in the viewpoint of the regulating bodies." With regards to medical doctors providing complementary care, he states that the guidelines are vague.

A practice within the regulating bodies that seems to be extremely inequitable is the fact that "conventional doctors are not required to inform patients of alternative [complementary] care available when offering conventional care. It does not go the other way around. When offering alternative medical care, I am required to tell the patient about the conventional care available for any given medical issue. I would like to know what the standard is—it is too vague. It's up to the viewpoint of the particular medical board."

This scenario is in part due to the fact that conventional medical schools emphasize disease management. A holistic physician believes that "in this day and age some form of minimal exposure to alternative medicine should be mandatory in medical schools because they need to know what their patients are getting in alternative care even if they do not offer it. If they don't know, they are ill informed. Some basic level of exposure should be mandatory in this day and age. The fact is that many people are using alternative medicine." He also notes that he would "like to see if they could upgrade education in the realms of diet and nutrition. Doctors don't know very much about diet. They just refer patients to the dietician. Nutrition is the fundamental basis of health, and more emphasis needs to be on it. There is increasing scientific evidence that this is true. More is being published."

Furthermore, an acupuncturist explained that the conventional system is "still geared to only care after illness or injury." Although preventive care is encouraged by the ACA, the act does not change the focus of disease management that pervades the current system. It is common knowledge that when people take responsibility for their health and live healthy lifestyles, there is decreased risk of disease. But little has changed in the current system to support this fact. Medical schools do a stellar job of teaching future doctors about disease but have very few mandatory courses educating doctors on how a healthy body works and is maintained.

It is common sense that if you want patients to take responsibility for their health and prevent diseases, doctors must know exactly what it takes to maintain a healthy body. The physicians I spoke to about this confirmed that there are only about thirty hours of nutrition taught in medical schools. There are elective courses, but they are not mandatory. That sends a clear message to providers to focus on disease. This focus is far more expensive than maintaining a healthy lifestyle.

As the acupuncturist said, "I see everything from chronic disease to mental health to physical injury to age-related issues—I see it across the board. If you got people to exercise and improve diet their whole life, they would still have some age-related issues and of course accidents do occur," but it would improve health overall. "This is still a disease-focused system—it's their game, it's their court, and their ball in the CPT coding system."

She continues, "In the government and in Congress, they [the conventional system] have huge lobbying efforts. The American Medical Association has no problems with influence—they have a strong voice with the government." This provider sees "the answers to this issue will come from people who are deciding to go into medicine to help others. There are also those who want to make money, of course."

As noted earlier, the CPT coding system is inadequate for the range of modalities needed to provide patients with the treatment options that each individual requires. Health care insurance companies generally follow the recommendations of the AMA or the conventional medical community when discerning what services are covered by insurance. Other than chiropractic and acupuncture, I do not know to what extent the determinations include complementary modalities, but from my experience and those I interviewed, complementary treatments are commonly not covered by medical insurance. And it was asserted repeatedly that most patients want complementary modalities covered by insurance.

Liability and malpractice are also constant concerns among many providers of health care, and they also become obstacles for giving the best care and keeping costs down. Often, providers feel the necessity to order additional tests "just in case" or feel pressured by patients to find the answers to their problems. This is a huge issue for providers and at times produces a very stressful environment for them. A physician shares this about end-of-life decisions: "A lot of overcare is fear of being sued. You need a legal document for the patient to say, 'I don't want it.' The same rules apply for babies—this is a very difficult situation. The hospitals do all these heroic things even for a baby who has no hope of living. A feeling for humanity is necessary."

Indeed, the great need for a more humanitarian health care system is a message I heard over and over. The current system based on profits and power lacks the humanity that creates a compassionate, caring, and effective system that provides patients with the tools they need to live healthy, happy lives.

We have much work to do to bring our health care system to this point. As individuals we can express our needs and desires to those in higher places and be assertive when we walk into a medical practitioner's office. We must educate ourselves and know our own bodies and our own individual needs. More providers of conventional care must make an effort to learn about the complementary/natural options of care—if not in medical school, from other professional sources. We must begin to take responsibility for the current state of affairs. It will not change until many of us do just that.

THE INFORMATION SUPERHIGHWAY

The Internet has changed our experience of the world. At the touch of a button, we can search for everything imaginable. There is almost nothing that has not been posted, written about, or documented in some way. This is both a blessing and a curse. Although there are many, many reputable websites, some are more reliable than others. And when you are searching for an accurate site for medical information, it can be challenging. Recently, I was referred to a website that is compiling all the recent scientific studies into a more user-friendly application. The website developer notes that a popular site, Medline, which can be accessed through public libraries, can be confusing and is not user friendly.

It is not within the scope of this book to discuss which sites are good and which are not. My point is that the information is out there to be discovered, and it is to the benefit of both patients and providers of care to understand the impact of this information and address it directly. It is not helpful for a physician to just dismiss an idea that a patient has painstakingly researched. The standard of care is narrow and needs to be made more flexible, but in the meantime we can improve relationships with our providers and have more open and satisfying dialogue if both parties are willing.

This is essentially a paradigm shift. This kind of interaction seldom exists in conventional medicine. It is not financially feasible within the context of the current insurance reimbursement system—the system does not support this type of partnership between patient and provider. In addition, most conventional providers are not educated in complementary medical care. However, that will change when the panels that create the standard of care begin to seriously examine the scientific data behind many complementary modalities and embrace those that show merit. And more and more patients need to pressure the system to include additional complementary modalities in the reimbursement process because many of these types of treatments improve the quality of life for patients.

Listening to patients who insist on partnering with their health care providers is quite encouraging in this respect. As a woman in her sixties states, "I want to participate in my health care. I will drop a doctor if he does not give me good care and shop for another one. I will try the care of my physician but do not see him as God. I will stop treatment if I think it is hurting me. I will speak up to my doctor and want a doctor who respects my opinion." This is an empowered woman.

And she is not alone. Many patients feel insulted and offended by a provider of care who refuses to think outside the box, especially when patients want to take responsibility for their own health and try options other than the standard of care. As one of the biggest complaints from conventional doctors is that their patients do not comply with treatment, they need to address the issue that there may just be a better way to treat a patient than the standard of care.

Because there are numerous scientific studies presented daily that offer real proof that complementary modalities show promise in a population of non-compliant patients, it behooves the professionals who decide on the standard of care to be more open to other treatments. The majority of complementary modalities has little or no side effects, unlike many of the new drugs presented to patients on a regular basis. Moreover, without the support of conventional medical providers, complementary medicine has and will continue to develop outside of the current system of medical care. That is not conducive to continuity of care, especially when there is a lack of mutual respect and openness among conventional and holistic practitioners.

Nearly all patients I interviewed preferred trying noninvasive techniques and commonsense treatment prior to drugs and procedures. Even if these treatments do not provide the results the provider wants to see, subsequently, the patient will likely be more willing to follow more invasive treatment instructions. As is reported by many patients, holistic treatments often help people feel better. A happy patient is a more compliant patient.

A registered nurse of many years shared stories of her experiences with patients. Many patients would not question the doctor, and as a nurse she would encourage them to ask questions. With all of her experience as a nurse, she believes that "most people should be one hundred percent involved in their health care and work together with the providers. People need to be aware of what goes on, what is good, and what is bad [for them]."

There is no question that patients who participate in their health in general have better outcomes. This mantra was repeated often in the interviews with patients. "I take responsibility for my health and participate in my care," states a middle-aged woman. She continues, "It is my body, and my outcomes have been mostly positive." These patients ask pertinent questions, pay attention to what works and doesn't work for them, and speak up to their providers when necessary.

A partnership between provider and patient can be a powerful combination. This is good for them as well as for the health care system as a whole.

Part Four

A Vision for Optimal Health Care

12

MIND-BODY MEDICINE AND THE STATUS QUO

The doctor of the future will give no medicine but will interest his patients in the care of the human frame, in diet, and in the cause and prevention of disease.

~ *THOMAS EDISON*

T HE BODY OF work that comprises scientific studies of the human body is as-tonishing. Technological advances allow us to investigate the most intricate systems that sustain life within us. Yet the more we learn, the more we realize we need to learn. Scientists have written volumes on how to manipulate this mysterious system, change or eliminate a symptom, or kill a disease or bacteria. Management of the body is the focus of conventional medicine—and the major focus is disease.

When I contemplate the reason for this, I realize that for centuries, entire populations were eliminated by certain diseases and plagues. The priority, of course, was to stop the massive deaths. It was necessary to focus on disease. We did not know enough about the human body, nor did we have the technology to see deeply into cells and tissues.

Although there were healers over time who intuited something at work in the human body other than what could be seen with the naked eye, this knowledge and wisdom eventually was left by the wayside when scientific discoveries of the causes of diseases and the mechanisms of the body hurled the healing profession into management of disease and systems within the human frame. The wisdom and knowledge that had been discovered naturally and intuitively by ancient societies became old school, and whether through hubris or enthusiasm or a combination of both, physicians and health practitioners concentrated more on the body rather than the person as a whole.

This perception of healing is disconcerting to most sick people, who are in need of a compassionate, caring human being to support them in their illnesses. In a world heavily connected by technology, people need real connections with other people. This is who we are. We are not machines to be repaired.

Mind-body medicine is deeply ingrained in the healing profession as a whole. From psychotherapy to integrative medicine, many practitioners understand the impact of the mind on the body. There are volumes of research on the subject. It is not new. In fact, the placebo effect has been proven in scientific studies to be 80 percent effective—more effective than most conventional therapies.

Psychologist Daniel Goleman, PhD, compiled a book on the subject entitled *Mind Body Medicine*. It addresses the power of meditation—a practice that has been studied extensively—as well as studies on visualization that helped cancer patients in Cleveland Hospital.

Dr. David Spiegel, a psychiatrist at Stanford University, ran support groups for terminal cancer patients, created for the sole reason of emotional support. The unintended consequence was that this group lived longer than those without the support (Goleman 1993, 3–4).

This knowledge resulted in much research being done to prove the mind-body connection—that our minds, thoughts, and emotions affect our physical health. This is a basic principle of mind-body medicine. It suggests the importance of patient involvement and the need for the practitioner of care to address emotional stress as well as physical stress in the standard of care. In spite of the research that has been available, conventional medicine has not fully embraced the mind-body connection.

The connection between the brain and immune system was also studied, revealing the connection between the central nervous system (CNS) and the immune system. This created the new field of psychoneuroimmunology.

Four major universities worked on research of mind-body medicine: Harvard University, Duke University, the University of California, and the University of Miami. Clinical studies suggested a strong correlation between our mental status and overall health. There were three levels of study: physical, psychological, and clinical testing. The clinical testing addressed the correlation between the use of mind-body medicine and relieving, managing, or preventing illnesses and diseases. (Goleman 1993, 5–10).

The authors also suggest that partnerships between providers of care and patients in modern medicine, although challenging, would bring back a more caring attitude and encourage patients to be involved in their healing processes.

There is very strong evidence that mind-body medicine is able to support sick patients in acquiring a better quality of life. There are several reasons to integrate mind-body medicine into mainstream medicine: the risks are low to zero, it is cost effective, and it can be used along with conventional medicine (Goleman 1993, 10–18).

Dr. Luskin and Dr. Pelletier's book, *Stress Free for Good*, is based on scientifically proven life skills that reduce stress. These studies, done at Stanford University, revealed repeatedly how important the mind is in reducing physical stress reactions. As an example, the skills include breathing techniques but also include the skill of appreciation—"noticing the good in your life" (Pelletier 2005, 63, 75).

In his book *The Instinct to Heal,* psychiatrist Dr. David Servan-Schreiber notes research on emotional support in patients, observing that "optimal functioning depends on relations with others," especially those we love. He argues that even though there is substantial scientific evidence to back the importance of relationships as affecting us physiologically, this important aspect of health is not readily accepted as valid in mainstream medicine. He remarks that procedures, medical equipment, and drugs can be patented, but relationships cannot (Servan-Schreiber 2004).

It is time for mainstream medicine to expand its perception of health care in the United States. As Dr. Albert Schweitzer is quoted as saying, "Every patient carries her or his own doctor inside."

There is a significant amount of brain research being done today, and I believe that it will eventually prove the mind-body connection more completely. My hope is that conventional medicine will integrate these findings into its standard of care.

THE OLD AND THE NEW

I have observed that when scientists make a new, exciting discovery, they stand firmly rooted in the new discovery and find the old outdated. They often throw aside the old as if it has little value, as if it could not possibly stand up to the greatness of their new findings. That has caused some serious repercussions. For example, I was born at a time when mothers' milk was thought to be inferior to what food scientists created for nourishment for babies. In the 1970s and 1980s when I had children, it was still not encouraged. I did nurse and was happy that I did, but I was basically on my own. Assistance in the hospital was minimal. The La Leche League was the only group that supported new mothers in this way, and I contacted them independently of my doctor or hospital.

Today, that seems rather ludicrous, but that trend lasted for decades. We now acknowledge that nature has supplied the perfect sustenance for each new baby and that encouraging the mother to nourish herself during pregnancy is the best assurance for proper nourishment for her offspring.

Another scientifically backed belief in the 1970s and 1980s was that margarine was a much better food than butter. Saturated fats were considered to be the enemy (and in some ways still are). Then thirty-five to forty years later, it was discovered that the very substance that was touted as healthy was contributing to heart disease. Trans fats present in margarine and in many processed foods were a real problem.

Moreover, it is important to note that due to the food industry's lobbying efforts, currently an item in the grocery can be labeled as "zero trans fats" even when it contains a small amount of it. The issue that I have with this regulation is that a person who eats a large quantity of processed food may end up ingesting a substantial amount of trans fats without knowing it.

Another trend beginning in the 1990s has found authoritative approval. The government and other authorities such as the American Medical Association are promising Americans that genetically modified foods (GMOs) are safe. The industry is fighting every grassroots group around the country who tries to pass a law to have foods containing GMOs labeled. Using fear tactics, these corporations are spending millions upon millions of dollars to discourage consumers from allowing such a law. As I stated earlier, the corporations like Monsanto, who manufacture and make huge profits from the use of GMOs, are the ones who are responsible for most of the studies that "prove" that GMOs are safe. That is a huge conflict of interest. The studies cannot be trusted.

Furthermore, there are independent studies that show GMOs are not safe. To me and to many other educated consumers, injecting toxins that kill insects into the DNA of a seed seems counter to producing health. The government has the responsibility to consumers to have these items labeled. If people want to consume them, that is certainly their choice, but we who do not want to consume them have the right to avoid them as well.

In addition, the farmers who use the GMO seeds must purchase them every year. It is a patented product and cannot be reused. This is a burden to many farmers and threatens organic farming when seeds wander and spread. For more information on genetically modified organisms, you can go to the WebMD website, which has an article that addresses the pros and cons ("The Truth about GMOs" 2015).

It could take decades for the effects on human health to become clear and to become public knowledge. In the meantime, it is prudent to allow individuals to decide for themselves. Like most other ingredients in food, GMOs need to be labeled.

I perceive the entire issue of safety from a much different angle from the governments and the powers that be. I would like for the corporations to prove the safety of an item utilizing longitudinal studies before it is put on the market, instead of allowing people to be the testing ground for safety. This includes the use of chemicals and additives in foods and in the environment.

There are tens of thousands of chemicals and additives in use in our country, and only about seven hundred or so have been thoroughly tested. In many cases, it is the burden of the consumer to prove the product unsafe. Thus we have many grassroots organizations that attempt to level the playing field in politics by giving the public a voice.

One other example of a popular treatment today in conventional medical is statins for high cholesterol. By their standards, it is one of the best ways to lower the risk of heart disease. It is considered to be an essential part of preventive medicine. And in some cases, drugs appear to be the only things that reduce high cholesterol—but in a very small number of people. In ten years from now, if the use of statins as standard of care is found not to be the magic bullet it was promised to be, the repercussions could be serious.

The point I am attempting to convey is that the human body is so complex that it behooves scientists to be more cautious about claims that may not stand up to the test of time, especially when the treatments have the potential of having serious side effects. Some of these effects, however, do not surface immediately—it takes time.

What is confusing to many patients is the degree of certainly with which the conventional medical community and other government and authoritative groups tout some of these new discoveries as absolute truth. For decades, eating margarine was considered to be essential for good heart health, and it was absolutely false.

Many medical treatments are meant to treat symptoms and do not change what is causing the imbalance in the body. Yes, a treatment or drug may take away the symptom, but that does not solve the real issue. What is causing the symptom? Conventional medicine may not have any other treatment to offer and often tells the patient they must live with the issue. I do not believe that is compassionate health care. For many patients, this treatment is not acceptable, and that view is becoming more and more common—thus, the increase in patients using complementary methods of healing.

Patients deserve to be partners in care and have other options than drugs and quick fixes. If conventional medicine does not have them, it is patients' responsibilities to become aware of other practitioners to provide care in different ways. It is doctors' responsibilities to make that known to their patients. This is about respect for the patient. Let the patient decide—it is their right.

The patriarchal system of health care is coming to an end. Patients want to be partners in their health care, not just be told what to do. Many providers want a system that respects their needs and provides better care to their patients. Change is difficult for everyone.

13

A COOPERATIVE SYSTEM OF CARE

Coming together is a beginning; keeping together is progress; working together is success.

~HENRY FORD

THE UNITED STATES is torn. As a society, we have fallen into a deep hole. We have bought into the us-against-them mentality, the "me generation," and most of all, we have forgotten that we are all in this together. The great United States is in discord.

Our communities are fragmented and driven by a multitude of private interests. Society is experiencing a split in perception that is deeply painful. Cooperating to create a path of action that results in the common good is our greatest challenge. That pertains to health care as well.

With regards to this system, there is hope in the number of professionals and interest groups exhibiting innovation and creativity in thought. There are many new organizations emerging and books penned by physicians and other professionals within recent years that question the effectiveness and, in some cases, the morality of the current system and the path we are presently on.

In the book *The Uncertain Art* by Dr. Sherwin Nuland, professor of surgery at Yale University, the wisdom of the biotech revolution in cloning of animals and eventually humans is questioned. He likens our society to "an overstimulated child" who does what he likes and what makes him happy without understanding the ramifications of his actions (Nuland 2008, 15).

Dr. Nuland also proposes that the standard that Western medicine uses to validate treatment could be reexamined. In acupuncture, there is significant evidence to prove that it works in many areas of illness and even in the operating room. Although it has thousands of years of successful use, conventional medicine has been unable to prove its effectiveness through the current scientific method. He suggests that there is sufficient proof from other methods of analysis and that a change in perspective may be in order (Nuland 2008, 58). Furthermore, he acknowledges the mind-body connection, placebo effect, emotional effects of various individuals on their diseases, and spontaneous remission. He is aware that the healings confound the scientific mind, yet he does not dismiss them but rather affirms them (Nuland 2008, 105–107).

Another book I recommend is *Better* by Dr. Atul Gawande, also the author of the new book *Being Mortal*. In *Better,* Dr. Gawande addresses issues such as going beyond the standard of care and following your intuition when treating a patient, as well as the problem of trying to fix a dying patient by always doing more. His emphasis is on what is right for an individual patient. The book contains many stories of patient care that provide teachable moments (Gawande 2007).

Dr. Sandeep Jauhar, author of *Doctored*, candidly responds to the values in medicine today. He addresses the power and profits that he believes allow doctors' values to change, allowing them to be part of the problem in the current system of health care. Dr. Jauhar admits that doctors are not always honest with their patients, especially when they make a mistake. He believes most of them believe the US health care system is the best, even when there is substantial proof that this is not the case. However, he does believe that medical students have the best chance of changing the system because they have fewer expectations (Jauhar 2014, 209, 257).

On the positive side, Medicare is considering compensating hospitals for better outcomes and fewer readmissions, and Dr. Jauhar sees that as optimistic. Although, he submits that this consideration is unbalanced and thinks that doctors also need to be rewarded for good care (Jauhar 2014, 228–229).

PATIENT-CENTERED CARE

In addition to professionals speaking out in books, there are organizations working to create a better system. The current system sees an imbalance and is working toward more patient-centered care. But patient-centered care will take time. We don't expect that all providers of care will immediately become great listeners, nor do we expect that patients will decide to speak up in their providers' offices because they know they can. It is a process, one that requires education on the part of patients and practitioners, as well as policy changes.

A partnership process between patients and doctors is slowly being integrated into our current system of health care. In this scenario, doctors must become familiar with not only the medical history, but the lifestyle circumstances that are a part of an individual's experience. It becomes imperative for patients to learn how to be more assertive, more independent in self-care, and more knowledgeable of their own bodies. When one considers the myriad of personalities and issues, it is clear that this is truly a paradigm shift.

Regarding this type of system, there is some concern that patients don't always know what is best for them. Yet in a patient-centered system, respect for patients' desires must be paramount. As I mentioned before, the patriarchal system of health care is changing, and the new paradigm is emerging. Although men continue to run many large organizations, that is changing more every day, especially in health care, where so many women are practitioners. Providers are less and less perceived as godlike and infallible. Patients are beginning to see their doctors and providers as people like them. They respect their providers' opinions, but many patients will no longer blindly submit to medical treatment. More often patients are not expecting to be fixed by their practitioners but realize the importance of their participation in the process. I predict this will only increase over time. As more patients learn how to clarify their situations, get to know and pay attention to the needs of their individual bodies, and take responsibility for their health while improving their health outcomes, it will open the door for truly effective and caring relationships between patients and providers.

Good communication is a skill and, when necessary, must be taught and nurtured in our current health care system. It can make the difference between success and failure. We are always in relationships with others, whether it be at home, at work, or in a medical office. Making good connections and building trust between patients and providers can only improve a troubled system.

To reiterate what I've said before, good communication between providers of care is also an essential component in improving the fragmented health care system. Better communication between practitioners caring for the same patient will enable each health care provider to be more informed, and the patient will receive better overall care. According to the people I interviewed, both patients and providers, this communication is lacking and, in the worst-case scenarios, results in medical errors.

As the younger generation moves into the system, they enter with new and different perspectives. This will help to move the system forward. It then becomes critical for the institutions of learning to immediately reflect changes of the new perspective into their medical school curriculum. It also would be to the providers' benefit for hospitals and other organizations to offer required workshops and webinars to engage the practicing providers in the patient-centered transition.

Empowered Patients

Another positive action is to create a system where patients have the opportunity to be educated and coached with respect to taking responsibility for their health. When education is provided and self-responsibility is rewarded by insurance companies, as it is in today's wellness programs offered by some employers, motivation on the part of the patient increases. This has resulted in fewer insurance claims and lower premiums, as I can attest to because of a family member's experience with their employer-provided wellness program. I also experienced this as a consultant with two of these wellness companies. Patients are being rewarded for educating themselves and taking preventive steps regarding their health. That is a step in the right direction.

Empowered patients take honest looks at their health, their outcomes, and the paths that led them to their health statuses. A helpless or victim attitude is not useful and will not provide motivation for change. Instead, creating a partnership with their provider or health coach with open, honest communication will support individuals in moving forward.

Doing your homework as a patient is essential as well. Get to really know your body, pay attention to your lifestyle, seek out supportive people in your life, and ask for feedback. Do your own research. Educate yourself about your illness, and seek out competent experts in both conventional and holistic medicine. Talk to friends and family, and find a caring and skilled provider. Choose a different doctor or practitioner if you are not happy with the one you have. Get a second or even third opinion when dealing with a confusing or serious illness. It is your body and your life.

There are numerous books available that afford patients helpful, empowering information. One that I like is *The Take-Charge Patient: How You Can Get the Best Medical Care* by Martine Ehrenclou. It contains some very valuable information and tips. There are also many websites that are supportive in creating a path to great health. Moreover, there are many computer programs and apps that you can purchase that provide reminders, tips, and other elements to keep a patient on track while he or she learns to take responsibility for his or her own health. For those who need support, this is a great place to start.

Patient advocacy must be considered when contemplating patient empowerment. Some of my interviewees were very strong on this issue, especially those who had experienced a serious illness and were hospitalized. When you as a patient are unconscious or unable to speak for yourself, it is very helpful to have a family member or friend who is authorized to speak for you. Be certain that the paperwork for this support is in place. A medical directive is necessary in a case where a patient cannot make his or her own decisions. Choose someone who is straightforward, assertive, and capable of following through on your personal wishes regarding health care decisions. Mistakes do happen, and a family member or friend overseeing care is extremely helpful, especially in a system under stress.

It is equally important and helpful to name a spokesperson or have one available on a doctor's visit in which important decisions are being made. It is difficult at times to keep a clear head when receiving bad news. Someone who will document the visit and instructions is beneficial. Documenting and tracking health history and treatment plans, obtaining medical records, and asking the provider for clarity and additional options are steps one can take to become an empowered patient.

Finally, remember to stay engaged in your own health, get regular checkups, maintain a diet that is healthy for you as an individual, and choose an exercise program tailored for your needs. We are all different, and what is good for your neighbor or even your sister or brother may not work well for you. Prevention is much easier than healing from an illness. Do what is right for you.

14

THE EVOLUTION OF MEDICINE

Education is the most powerful weapon which you can use to change the world.

~NELSON MANDELA

WHAT IS OUR focus on when we consider our health? Is it the absence of disease or the infusion of life? What does it mean to have a well-functioning body and mind? I believe that the more we know about a well-functioning body and mind, the healthier we will all be. I do not place the most value in health care on sickness and what might be wrong, but on how I can optimize the wonders of this body of mine. I believe it is prudent and common sense to consider that good health care can be based on what a healthy body is as well as the study of disease.

Unfortunately, like much of life, conventional medicine focuses on what is wrong with our body and not what is right. Yes, it does celebrate good health and encourage preventive screenings, but most of the money for research goes toward finding cures, studying the science of diseases, and discovering how to fix them or manipulate symptoms of the body. The war against disease is much like the war on drugs, and neither has been truly successful. People are living longer and are saved from death more often, but the quality of life on many medications and while living with chronic diseases is far from optimal.

The human body is a miracle. Yet with all of the science, there is still so much we don't know. Furthermore, no two patients react the same to treatments. It takes great skill to learn what is good for one patient over another. Much of that skill is learned primarily with experience and continuing education. It is interesting to note that scientists who study the universe know their limitations with regards to knowledge and understanding. However, often in conventional medicine, we as patients and practitioners are expected to trust the science implicitly without questioning it. What is lacking in medical research are studies that help us to understand, respect, and work with the human body and its innate systems of homeostasis and healing.

It confounds me that Western medicine refuses to utilize the evidence-based complementary modalities that have eliminated so much suffering and achieved success with so many patients, while at the same time making little effort to learn about these modalities. I wonder how different things would be if medical schools would make that knowledge mandatory, at least in part. In my research, I found some evidence that CAM is being taken seriously by mainstream medicine. The system that holds the power has the financial means to do more research. However, most of the research is still dedicated to studying disease and looking for cures, further supporting a disease-focused system.

This is unfortunate and does not sit well with the patients I spoke with. They see a closed system unwilling to open its mind to other possible ways of healing. I have heard over and over again from doctors and other mainstream practitioners that patient compliance is often unsatisfactory. They wonder how they can get their patients to be more compliant. When more patients are respected, given balanced options, and provided the support and education they need to improve their lifestyles, they will be more compliant, and our health outcomes will improve immensely.

Patients and practitioners want honesty, but the honesty must be on both sides of the equation. Providers of care need to say when they don't know what is wrong or don't know about other options. It is their responsibility to take some time to learn the basics about well-known modalities that result in positive outcomes for their patients. They need to know a CAM provider to refer their patients to when appropriate, and it would follow that they need to relate in a positive way to CAM providers and work as a team. Patients are in great need of this type of relationship in their health care experiences.

I recently listened to a webinar from Canadian CBC radio in Ontario, Canada. The interviews were with patients as well as conventional providers of care. With regards to CAM, the usual arguments about lack of science were mentioned, as well as the need to integrate conventional and complementary medicine and have the best of both worlds. Canada's national health program relies on conventional practitioners to refer their patients for complementary treatments. That, of course, can be problematic. Even though CAM in Canada is more accepted than in the United States, it is still not fully integrated into the system.

Canada does regulate dietary supplements and other natural health care products and educates their citizenry as well. They are working to regulate chiropractic and naturopathic medicine. However, they have promised regulations and standards since 2007 without results (CBC Radio Ontario 2014). I can imagine that politics is involved. Even though Canada is ahead in some ways, they also have a long way to go.

I interviewed a Canadian patient who complained about the disease-focused system of care in Canada and how things could be so much better. About conventional medicine, he laments:

> There is no one talking about how to make us well. Everything is the quick fix. The pharmaceutical companies keep providing the quick fixes, that fit with their mandate, and they are very profitable in doing so. Within the system there is very little motivation for change. I think what happens is that the patients think they don't have the power to make a difference. Yet, people are changing the system because they are going to alternative practitioners and reading more. But I believe that more people will be asking to look at the root cause. Then doctors

will be more interested, and those who don't look at root causes will lose patients. When more people learn that there are so many more options available, things will change more rapidly. It is a matter of time. In the meantime, we need to just try to make a difference. I think this is the same for Canada and probably most countries in the world. The system is driven by money, and disease is money. We need to find some ways to change from that perspective.

This patient does have complementary medicine providers that he is pleased with—some things are covered by their national program, and some are not. He says he doesn't get much pushback from his conventional doctors about CAM, but he does not believe they understand what he is doing. There are team systems set up in Canada, however, whose main purpose is to create a plan that works well for the patient and results in positive outcomes. The patient says that this system is fairly new and "can make a difference."

There is no doubt that optimal health care has a long way to go in the United States as well. Patients and providers have a stake in better health care outcomes. We need to consider a different perspective if we are to see better results and lower health care costs. What we are doing is not working. When all parties involved take responsibility for their part in a broken system, things will change.

The sense of separateness among the professionals in the health care field needs to evolve. Providers must become part of the solution and not just comply with the status quo. We all need to cooperate with valid systems of care. When I think of the potential of utilizing all of the knowledge of conventional medicine and CAM, it is exciting. We can use our creative minds and hearts and find the answers; we can change this broken system.

Consider the old saying "divide and conquer." Those (individuals and corporations) with power and money in our current system know full well that in order to maintain their power, they need to divide those they have power over. It behooves Big Pharma and huge corporations and foundations who are greatly invested in the status quo to feed arguments that will divide groups, creating fear of "the other". Imagine the power of practitioners utilizing the knowledge of disease in the body with those who understand what creates and maintains a healthy body. Our society would be far healthier and happier, and health care costs would substantially drop.

As a patient observes, "There is only one world out there. We are in this together."

It will take courage to create a new, more effective system of health care. Let's work together.

FORWARD-THINKING ORGANIZATIONS

As more and more people involved in the system look for resolution to our health care crisis, organizations are creating groups that educate and unite. This will evolve and grow. The following list is not all inclusive but is representative of the movement toward positive change.

One organization previously mentioned is the American Institute for Cancer Research. That group is taking the lead in researching and educating professionals and the public on how to lower their risk of cancers and how to get through a cancer experience in the healthiest way possible. They teach a healthy diet and lifestyle as powerful tools in this area.

The Center for Integrative Medicine at the University of Maryland School of Medicine evaluates CAM research studies and provides education to the public as well as to professionals. It is also involved in "integrating evidence-based complementary therapies into clinical care to help people achieve and maintain optimal health and well-being" (The Center for Integrative Medicine 2015).

In New York City, a group of forward-thinking health care practitioners and professionals has organized under the name of the Functional Forum. This new educational setting "brings together the latest health news, functional medicine research, practice development and health technology in an upbeat, entertaining way." It is open to all health care professionals, and they offer monthly online trainings and conferences (Functional Forum 2014).

On the health-coaching front, the Institute for Integrative Nutrition® is the largest school in the world that teaches nutrition. Their mission is to empower health coaches to bring health and happiness to the world. Their curriculum reveals holistic healing at its best (Institute for Integrative Nutrition

2015). Graduates are also members of The International Association for Health Coaches (IAHC) that advocates for health coaching all over the world (International Association for Health Coaches 2015).

The National Consortium for Credentialing of Health & Wellness Coaches, cofounded in 2009 by Wellcoaches® founder Margaret Moore, is in the process of creating training standards for health coaches and working to advance coaching research in academic medical establishments. Their mission is to integrate professional health and wellness coaches into the health care system, providing support to Americans struggling to maintain a healthy lifestyle (NCCHWC 2015).

The Green Road Project is a philanthropic partnership. One of the partners is Captain Fred Foote, MD, who worked as a military physician for twenty-nine years. He and others partnering with the Institute for Integrative Health in Baltimore, Maryland, brought to life the Green Road Project, which brings wounded warriors into nature to help them heal. There is evidence that a natural environment lowers stress and promotes healing, especially for those with conditions such as PTSD. This natural woodland area on the campus of Walter Reed National Military Medical Center offers wounded soldiers a place to visit with family, rest, and recuperate. It is free of traffic and is wheelchair accessible. Once the project is completed at the end of 2015, they will begin scientific research on the healing effects of the Green Road.

15

Optimal Health

*Although the world is full of suffering, it is also full of the
overcoming of it.*

~ Helen Keller

W HAT DOES OPTIMAL health mean to you? Most people would say that it
is everything—that without good health you have nothing. Yet in the
United States, many people choose lifestyles that make good health almost
impossible.

Merriam-Webster defines *health* as "the condition of being sound in body,
mind, or spirit; freedom from physical disease or pain." I would define *health* as
living life to the fullest in body, mind, and spirit.

Before I started a truly healthy lifestyle, I thought I was fine. I had my ups
and downs, but most of the time I felt all right. No complaints. Although, I
noticed that when my body felt better and my mind was peaceful, I was more
content. When my mood was good, my outlook on life was even better. Then I

started to pay attention and experiment with food, exercise, and spiritual practice. That is when I began to fully understand what optimal health is.

As a human being, I am part of the earth. I came from elements of the earth and from my mother's body, I depend on these elements in nature to sustain this body and mind, and I nurture my spirit with things that cannot be experienced with my senses alone. When I fill my life with stuff and mindless physical pleasures, giving no consideration to the value of this wonderful creation that carries me through life, and when I do not consider my whole being, I am very disappointed in the results.

When we value our bodies and our minds, we can make good choices. It is so important to understand the value of who we are innately—not what we do or how much money we make, but who we are and what we have to offer. We have all made disappointing decisions, but it is imperative to forgive ourselves, dust ourselves off, and start again. Bring yourself back to who you really are, what you truly want, and live that truth again. Be vigilant and courageous daily.

Every person has a baseline. When people decide to improve their overall health, they move forward from where they are. This experience is varied, and the tools that one person uses may not work for another. To know what good health is for you, it is essential to examine your life from a physical, emotional, spiritual, and social level while embracing your dreams and desires. We are complex creatures, but everyone has the need for sustenance, safety, and belonging.

Perceiving health in a more basic way is helpful when deciding what direction to take in life. When people consider those who do not have a home to live in or food to eat, their needs are simple—where do I sleep safely tonight, and where do I get something to eat? That becomes priority. No need to worry about friendship or a job—at least not at that point.

We live in a society that has an unbelievable amount of stuff. Stuff is not a necessity, but many of us spend so much of our lives collecting this stuff. It is a great diversion if we are trying to avoid other things in our lives. And for each person, those other things are different. Maybe we hate our jobs, have unhealthy relationships, or don't know what we want to do in life. I have found that when I identify something I really want to change or happen in my life, it gives me hope. If I then take a simple action toward it, I move closer to what I desire. But identifying what is important in my life is the first step in improving my overall health.

Optimal health varies and depends on your stage in life. We are all going to die. But we can feel good, empowered, and content on the journey. I don't believe for a minute that I am destined to feel achy, arthritic, bent over, or diseased. I feel that even though I have genes that may give me a tendency toward a certain disease, I don't have to acquire it. I don't have to turn the genes on. It is possible to override your genes and I do my very best to do that by making excellent lifestyle choices.

The study of Epigenetics deals with the behavior of genes and is a fascinating, fast-growing field of research. I hope this focus will become more integrated into conventional medicine. Integrating epigenetics into medical care has the capacity to empower both patients and providers and give hope to patients predisposed to certain diseases.

Attitude is so important too. I have a family member who is one hundred years old and recently had surgery. She went home the next day and feels fine. She has a wonderful, laid-back attitude on life and rolls with the punches. Although that is not my temperament, I strive in that direction, and I have greatly improved.

If I could give one piece of advice to everyone, it would be this: if you want optimal health, begin by knowing your body, your mind, and your spirit. Know yourself, and don't depend on anyone else to do that for you. Ask for support, yes. Do your research, yes. Do your work, yes. But always be at the helm when making important lifestyle changes. Seek your own wisdom—that still, small voice within each and every one of us.

One of the most important life lessons I have learned in my personal work and in my health-coaching work is that at some level, all people know what they need to do and what changes they need to improve their lives and their places in the world. Often, it takes self-examination, time, and patience to become aware of it. It takes surrounding yourself with people who are encouraging and supportive. It takes motivation and commitment to yourself.

Our journeys may be similar, but we are all unique and bring to life something very special. If we are homeless, our jobs on any given day may be to remain hopeful, ask for and receive what we need, and allow other people to experience the joy of giving to us. If we have everything we need, our jobs may be to show enthusiasm, to hold up and support others. The wonderful thing is that every day is a new beginning, and we can start again. This knowledge and having a purpose are as important as all the healthy lifestyle changes we can imagine.

Life is finite. We will not live forever. In fact, we have no idea how many more days of life we have here on Earth. That makes each day a gift and each moment special. Every person that we come face-to-face with every day provides us with an opportunity—to live. Every choice makes ripples in the fabric of life. We do not live in a vacuum. What we do and what we think affects others in one way or another.

We are not just bodies attempting to have better lives. We are human beings with needs and desires and something to contribute. When we as patients or practitioners meet one another, it is not just business as usual. We show up with our own special circumstances, moods, and skills. If we as patients or providers would just take deep breaths and really see the person in front of us, whether we agree with him or her or not, it is possible that honest, open communication would ensue. That in and of itself creates enormous potential in any situation.

Optimal health and optimal health care for both patients and providers can only exist in an environment of open, honest communication. Any system that operates on money and competition with a competition-based fear mentality cannot create a positive, healing environment. We must find a way to embrace our values and provide the finest health care system in the world. America is capable of this. Our culture of freedom and innovation makes this possible.

As participants in the health care system, we are all responsible for bringing it our best and taking steps that we see as important. As patients we can learn to be assertive, take responsibility for our health, and tell the truth to ourselves and our providers of care. As providers we can open ourselves to new knowledge, learn to listen, appreciate the wisdom of the body, tell the truth, and provide healing environments for patients.

Everyone who is part of this system has the responsibility to speak up for what is right and true. We must not be passive and accept the status quo. We, as individuals with our own unique strengths, are more powerful than that. We have the capacity to choose courage over fear, one step at a time. Every voice is important and needs to be heard. Remember the ripples—we all make ripples in our lives, no matter who or where we are. We all matter.

As my journey writing this book comes to an end, I feel humbled by all of the generous patients and practitioners I spoke with, all of the lessons I've learned as a giver and receiver of care, all the amazing opportunities that life has afforded me, and all the tremendous potential of human beings working to create a better health care system.

Look deeply within yourself and find the wisdom that can make all the difference in your life and in the lives of everyone you touch. The authentic self, who you really are—your best self—is the greatest contribution that you can make to our health care system and to the world.

AUTHOR BIOGRAPHY

JOAN LUSCO GUGERTY became interested in wellness and nutrition in the 1970s, when smoking was commonplace and only hippie communes talked about healthy eating.

Gugerty spent twenty years working in the health care field, mostly in administrative roles in hospitals, doctor's offices, and medical training facilities, giving her access to the entirety of conventional health care culture. She also worked for six years in a holistic physician's office and one year as a Health Coach in a physician's office.

In 2006-2008, Gugerty attended the Institute for Integrative Nutrition® in New York City, earning an integrative health coach certification, an experience that exposed her to leaders in the field of nutrition and integrative medicine. As a Wellness Consultant, she provides individual health coaching, motivational speaking, and wellness seminars to support people in living more healthy and peaceful lives. She is also the Founder and Director of Heartworks Wellness. The website is www.heartworkswellness.com.

Gugerty spent two years compiling information on patient and health provider experiences in the existing US health care system, which proved the catalyst for *Restoring Dignity.*

BIBLIOGRAPHY

2015. https://www.functionalmedicine.org.

2013. http://www.iom.edu.

2014. August 27. www.ips-dc.org.

2007. http://medicalnewswire.com/artman/publish/article_9539.shtml.

2015. http://www.compmed.umm.edu/default.asp.

2015. *ABC Coding Solutions.* http://www.abccodes.com/ali/faqs/general_faq. asp.

2015. *American College for Advancement in Medicine.* April. Accessed April 2015. http://www.acam.org.

Brill, Steve. 2015. *"America's Bitter Pill." In America's Bitter Pill*, by Steve Brill. New York: Random House.

2014. *CBC Radio Ontario.* December. Accessed 2014. http://www.cbc.ca/ontariotoday/index.html.

2013. *Center for Disiease Control.* www.cdc.org.

1993. In *Mind-Body Medicine*, by Ph.D and Joel Gurin, Editors Daniel Goleman, 3-4. Yonkers, NY: Consumers Union of United States.

2004. In *The Instinct to Heal*, by M.D., Ph.D David Serven Schreiber, 169. New York, NY: Rodale, Inc.

2014. *Functional Forum.* December. http://functionalforum.com/about.

2007. In *Better*, by Atul Gawande. Picador: New York, NY.

2015. *Institute for Integrative Nutrition.* April. Accessed April 2015. http://www. integrativenutrition.com/.

2015. *International Association for Health Coaches.* April. Accessed April 4, 2015. https://www.iahcnow.org/.

2015. *Medical Coding.* https://www.aapc.com/resources/medical-coding/icd9.aspx.

2015. *NCCHWC.* Accessed 2015. http://ncchwc.org.

2008. In *The Uncertain Art*, by Sherwin B. Nuland. New York, NY: Random House, Inc.

Parker, Steve. 2013. *Kill or Cure, Ann Illustrated history of Medicine.* New York, NY: Dorling Kindersley Limited.

2005. In *Stress Free for Good*, by Dr. Fred Luskin and Dr. Kenneth R. Pelletier, 63, 75. New York, NY: HarperCollins Publishers.

Potter, Wendell. 2010. *Deadly Spin.* New York, NY: Bloomsbury Press.

2002. *Public Broadcasting System.* http://www.pbs.org/healthcarecrisis/ history.htm.

2014. In *Doctored*, by M.D. Sandeep Jauhar.

Taylor, Elizabeth H. Bradley and Lauren A. 2013. *The American Health Care Paradox.* New York, NY: Public Affairs.

2015. *The Truth About GMOs.* http://www.webmd.com/food-recipes/features/ truth-about-gmos.

www.ingramcontent.com/pod-product-compliance
Lightning Source LLC
Chambersburg PA
CBHW070657290526
45790CB00001B/359